MOTHERHOOD

SMOTHERHOOD

MOTHERHOOD SMOTHERHOOD

Fighting Back Against the Lactivists,
Mompetitions, Germophobes,
and So-Called
Experts Who Are Driving Us Crazy

JJ Keith

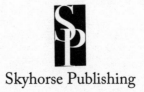

Skyhorse Publishing

Parts of this book have been adapted from the author's blogs, www.blogspot.jjustkidding.com *and* www.jjkeith.net *(the Versus Series), or were previously published on* www.babble.com *and* www.huffingtonpost.com.

Skyhorse Publishing books may be purchased in bulk at special discounts for sales promotion, corporate gifts, fund-raising, or educational purposes. Special editions can also be created to specifications. For details, contact the Special Sales Department, Skyhorse Publishing, 307 West 36th Street, 11th Floor, New York, NY 10018 or info@skyhorsepublishing.com.

Skyhorse® and Skyhorse Publishing® are registered trademarks of Skyhorse Publishing, Inc.®, a Delaware corporation.

Visit our website at www.skyhorsepublishing.com.

10 9 8 7 6 5 4 3 2 1

Library of Congress Cataloging-in-Publication Data is available on file.

Cover design by Brian Peterson
Cover photo credit Alden and JJ Keith

Print ISBN: 978-1-62914-658-4
Ebook ISBN: 978-1-63220-052-5

Printed in the United States of America

Praise for JJ Keith and *Motherhood Smotherhood*

"JJ Keith's writing is exceptionally gutsy, sometimes heartbreaking and always laugh out loud funny. She's the queen of finding a fresh angle on every topic. What I'm saying is, I'm jealous of her ability. Okay? There. The secret is out."

—Stefanie Wilder-Taylor, bestselling author of *Sippy Cups Are Not for Chardonnay and Naptime is the New Happy Hour*

"I love her stuff."

—Jenny Lawson (The Bloggess), *New York Times* bestselling author of *Let's Pretend This Never Happened*

"DUDE. This is epic. Every new mom needs a copy of *Motherhood Smotherhood*."

—Rebecca Woolf (Girls Gone Child), author of *Rockabye: From Wild to Child*

"JJ Keith's entertaining book succeeds where so many writers on parenting fail: she takes her experience, avoids universalizing it, and uses it to bring parents together, away from the myth of perfection parenting. *Motherhood Smotherhood* is filled with worldly perspective and an original voice. In short, it's frank, fresh, and funny. I wish I'd written it."

—Leanne Shirtliffe, author of *Don't Lick the Minivan: And Other Things I Never Thought I'd Say to My Kids*

"If for some reason I end up with a kid, this is the shit I would read."

—Samantha Irby (Bitches Gotta Eat), author of *Meaty: Essays*

"In today's culture of parenting do's and don'ts, those who seek out the 'best' child-rearing philosophies are often met with more questions than answers. JJ Keith demystifies those questions by asserting that no parent is perfect—and that's okay. Her relatable and witty essays soothe rather than worry, and for someone who's embarking on the parenting journey, that's the only advice that will really matter."

—Blair Koenig, author of *STFU, Parents: The Jaw-Dropping, Self-Indulgent, and Occasionally Rage-Inducing World of Parent Overshare*

"I should have written this. My bad."

—Dr. Benjamin M. Spock (posthumously via a reputable psychic)

For Alden,
The Leela to my Fry, the Larry to my Balky Bartokomous, and the
Shining Armor to my Princess Mi Amore Cadenza.

CONTENTS

Within the span of a few weeks, two pregnant friends approached me for advice about childbirth, breastfeeding, and taking care of a baby. I didn't know what to say. I mean, what do I know? I'm no expert. Try not to drop the baby? Don't forget to change the baby's diaper every few hours? Find a wooden spoon and bite on it until the baby turns one?

I muttered something like, "Uh, you don't need a stroller, but it's nice to have one? And, uh, definitely get a car seat. Swaddle, I think, if it works. It's like wrapping a burrito. Eh, Google it." My friends nodded along, kindly pretending that I was helpful. One of them asked me about books, and all I could come up with was, "Uh, anything but *Baby Wise*?" referring to the rigorously sched-uled technique that has caused some parents to undernourish their newborns and thus is no longer recommended by pediatricians.

Now that my kids were in preschool, all that baby stuff seemed far away and my "smell ya later, infancy" attitude wasn't helpful to my pregnant friends who wanted my advice. At some point after the second visit from a soon-to-be new mom, I drank about elev-enty beers and gave it some thought. The resulting "advice" went viral, first on my personal blog, and then the *Huffington Post*. Turns out that in between the attachment parenting zealots and sleep training fascists, there are a bunch of people whose attitudes are like mine: I just do shit and shit happens; I try not to be a dick to my kids, but it's okay if sometimes they're inconvenienced by my need to be a human in addition to being a mother.

The vast majority of chatter surrounding parenthood is junk. All of these seemingly divisive decisions—like pain meds in labor, newborn sleep arrangements, and scheduling—are often phrased as moral imperatives from both sides. Screw that. Take care of your kid. Do what works. Babies are more durable than we give them credit for. As a parent, I can be wrong as long as I realize it and change. That means it's okay to make educated guesses and then sort out the consequences. And it means I have to play this parenting gig by ear, which is disquieting for people with controlling tendencies like me. But I must control my tendency to be controlling or else I will imprison myself. Infants cannot be micromanaged, nor can toddlers, children, teenagers, spouses, or nannies. Parents who want to be perfect can knock themselves out, but I'd rather they not blame the institution of parenthood (or worse, their babies) when they go two years without finishing a sentence, sleeping through the night, or having sex.

My parenting philosophy can be summed up by the question, "Really?!" taken from the *Saturday Night Live* Weekend Update segment from the mid-aughts. It's how you should respond to the moms in your playgroup who tell you either "Ferberizing is the only way to go" or "Sleep training causes brain damage." And "Really?!" is the only acceptable response to a partner who claims "I don't know how to change diapers as well as you." But more than that, "Really?!" is the appropriately calm response to the old lady who scolds you to put a sweater on your baby in Trader Joe's on a swelteringly hot day, the young couple who gives you the stink eye when you walk into a restaurant with your baby, or the grand-parent who feels the need to point out that your newborn's outfit doesn't match. Blowing off random comments is far better than getting all huffy.

Once babies are born, parents have to know their enemies, but more importantly, they have to recognize that most people aren't their enemies. For every asshole sneering while Baby is wailing in the checkout line, there's another person behind them making funny faces to distract Baby. Parents choose where their focus goes: the funny-face person or the asshole, but this parenting stuff is hard enough without having to feel like the world is piling up on you. Let's give everyone else some credit, okay?

In later conversations with my pregnant friends, I clarified my advice. One of my favorite tips for new parents is to ask only a few friends for guidance, preferably those who are a kid or two ahead because they are ones who best understand that every baby is different—a vital component of good parenting advice. The rea-son that some techniques are beloved by some parents and reviled by others is that they work on some babies and not on others. Some babies exhaust themselves by crying and will only pass out after a good sob, while others get more amped up by crying and will go for hours. Some babies need to be held close all the time as prescribed by attachment parenting manuals, but some babies long for more independence and will push against a parent trying to force 24–7 closeness. Some babies want solid food when they're five months old, some will still be disinterested at ten months.

Nobody knows what kind of baby they have until they feel it out and make some mistakes. Plus, those little nuggets drift in and out of phases so quickly that it may seem like some baby care advice worked when, in fact, the kidlet coincidentally started sleeping through the night at the same time as a new sleep program was implemented. They are wildly unpredictable creatures, these babies of ours. And a large part of what makes them maddening is that they are so lousy at giving feedback. You know you've lost your mind when you plead with a four-month-old to "use your words." And yes, I'm saying that from experience. (And yes, I'm doing much better now that he's a toddler and has some words to use.)

And hey, you got yourself a baby. Lucky you! No really, lucky you. Who's the tickle monster? You're the tickle monster now! So sack up and have some fun with that little squirt.

THE WORLD'S SLOWEST
DEVELOPING POLAROIDS

Immediately after my daughter was born in 2009, I was inundated with advice (most of it contradictory or useless). I had my neighbor telling me to let my baby cry it out two days after I brought her home from the hospital. My mom was telling me to "never wake a sleeping baby," though my particular sleeping baby weighed five-and-a-half pounds and was shrinking rapidly because she was snoozing through her feedings. There was the pediatrician who pushed formula samples on me and the lactation consultant who instructed me to pump every three hours around the clock and feed my baby breast milk from a bottle. Then another mom admonished me, saying that breast milk in bottles is basically formula and another mother told me that formula was fast food for newborns.

As I settled into being a mom, I spent a lot of time reading parenting books and message boards. Little did I know that parenting boards are among the darkest and most pestilent trenches of the Internet; so awash with anxiety, judgment, and pointless debate about baby kneepads—are they a reasonable safety precaution or evidence of pathological overprotection? Who the fuck cares!— that I could hardly stand to venture there for simple advice on the benefits of acetaminophen versus ibuprofen lest I get sucked asunder into some debate about the efficacy of teething tablets versus a whisky-dipped pinkie finger versus cranial-sacral therapy. There are the lactivists ("Would you feed your baby Skittles? Well, then why would you feed her formula?"), and the sleep schedule fanatics ("If you don't get your baby on a schedule in the first week home from the hospital, then say goodbye to sleep for the next year"). It's all a bit much.

And some parents out there in the world aren't any better than the pseudo–experts or the message board trolls, especially in the early days of parenting. During my daughter's first year, I heard some atrocious things come out the mouths of parents (including mine). I recall being in a new mom group and hearing another mother go off about a woman who *dared* to show up for a breastfeeding support class wearing earrings: "I mean, who has time to put on earrings when you just had a baby?! Like, oh, sorry, Newborn, I'm just going to put you down while I put on earrings." Another time, I heard a dad rant about lazy parents who let their kids eat from the cart while at the grocery store. As far as I'm concerned, giving a bored baby a banana so you can finish your shopping is good parenting. Bonus points if you pay for the banana. People rant about gross moms who prepare nibbles for their baby by biting off pieces of fruit and spitting it out onto a plate, but I'm pretty sure that once someone has passed through my vagina and drunk from my tit, I'm allowed to slobber on their food a bit. I mean, I *could* carry around a hand-cranked food processor in my diaper bag *or* I could do whatever is going to get shit done with the least hassle. There's a world of good information out there, but even more crap. New parents who want to filter all that information must be very judicious about Internet usage and the company they keep.

There isn't one right way to do *anything*, let alone parenting, and that is scary as hell, but it's also freeing. The only thing that works is figuring it out as the baby grows, which I know is maddening because it's not instructive. There aren't any simple answers. But hey, it's good preparation for parenting older children, the ones who can hold a conversation and have feelings, which might seem like a vacation to someone with a baby at home, but is just as perilous as wiping the ass of a squirming baby. Not that there isn't anything to look forward to. Generally by the time they're old enough to damage parents' psyches with their words, they can wipe their own asses, so there's that.

Parenting is an ever-changing cost-benefit analysis. It doesn't get easier, but it does get to be more fun. There's such joy in exposing kids to the world piece by piece. I've found particular pleasure in bringing my children into contact with zoos, marching bands, nature, and my favorite building (Griffith Observatory in Los Angeles, in case anyone is wondering). To see my children watch a parade? Even a stupid canned parade at Disneyland? Tears in my eyes, people. That shit is fucking majestic! I've cried during the following occasions: 1) Riding bumper cars with them for the first time, 2) Telling them that the Earth is round and that there's land on the other side of the ocean, 3) Revealing to them that their grandma is my mom, 4) Teaching them to stir brownie batter, 5) Breaking down that words are made from letters, 6) Taking them with me to vote, 7) Explaining that catalogs are books from which people can select and pay for goods that will then be delivered (might have just been hormonal for that last one).

I can't wait to see what kind of adults my kids become. They are slowly developing but captivating little Polaroids. Before I had kids, if anyone had told me that a two-decade-long story arc could be enthralling, I would have made fun of them, and probably rightfully so because what an obnoxious way to put it. But watching them grow up really is that great. I don't even care if one or both of them Alex P. Keatons me, which is a verb defined as, "The act of offspring gleefully rebuking their parents' values, often including taking opposing political or religious views; named for the mid-eighties sitcom character on *Family Ties* played by Michael J. Fox, who was a blazer-wearing Reaganite, much to the chagrin of his hippie-dippy parents."

But the dark side of the childhood-length cliffhanger is the worry. Some of it is inevitable, but I try to never forget what my dad taught me. He really, really, really, really wanted me to grow up to be a Rush Limbaugh-loving Olympic athlete who appreciated the music of Lynyrd Skynyrd. Alas, today he is disappointed on all fronts. I'd rather not open myself up for that kind of disappointment in my kids. They were born with personalities of their own, and I see it as my job to keep them safe, comfortable, and supported while they grow into the people they're going to be.

It's great that parenthood is broadly associated with tenderness because there are so many booboos to kiss, and I do love that side of the gig, but I have come to a more diverse understanding of parenthood. After surviving two infancies so close together (my kids are twenty months apart), I now associate rearing newborns and toddlers with parents who are *tough as fuck*. No lie, at this point I could leg-press two toddlers while changing a newborn's diaper. I go *hard* on parenting. Like a boss.

What makes a good parent isn't breastfeeding for exactly twelve months as prescribed by the World Health Organization or offering the exact right amount of tummy time. It's far more nebulous than all that. Here's my survey for worried parents of babies: Have you washed dishes this week? Are you currently on crystal meth? Do you routinely use a car seat? Yes, no, yes? Then it's gonna be okay. If not now, then eventually. Unless you think you might have postpartum depression. If that's the case, first get some help, *and then* it's going to be okay.

I'm not pretending that I was this relaxed from the outset. When my first was a newborn, I Googled before I did anything, mommy-blogged every detail of my daughter's life as if I were the very first person who had thought to do so, went to so many mommy groups that talking about poop started to feel like a job, wrung my hands about what other parents thought of me, and got up in arms about parents who were doing things differently. It is really, really, really hard not to be a dick when you're a new parent and I tip my hat to anyone who manages to avoid it. I certainly didn't.

But despite all that writhing around and trying to perfect mothering, one thing I will grant myself is that I took pleasure in the gig from the get–go, mostly because I went through so much trying to become a mom. Before finally having my daughter, I had three miscarriages, all in the first trimester, each more devastating than the last. When I finally took my baby home from the hospital, I felt like the luckiest lady in the world. Not long after, a friend who was continuing to struggle with fertility issues asked me if it was hard having a newborn, and I answered quite truthfully, knowing that she would understand, that no, taking care of a baby is much easier than not having a baby to take care of when one is wanted. Despite some rough patches here and there, being a parent is a pretty fucking awesome experience and my delight never wanes (except when it does . . . but then it comes back).

WHY, YES. THERE IS A PERSON LODGED IN MY ABDOMEN. THANKS FOR ASKING.

After a prenatal yoga class, still barefoot and sweaty, I found myself on the receiving end of a lecture from a fellow yogi: "It's none of your business if twins run in my family! As if the contents of my reproductive system are any concern of yours! They don't call them private parts for nothing!"

I'd meant my question innocently. When she told me she was having twins, I was excited. Two children + one tummy = mind-blowing! I was desperate to engage her and find out more about her super-sized pregnancy, but I see now that she probably thought I was trying to find out if she'd used reproductive technology to get pregnant, something I hear moms of twins are rudely asked about all the time.

I should have known better since I was having my own struggles with the curiosity of strangers. I found out I was pregnant again just after my firstborn turned one, or as one elderly gentleman on the street informed me, "too soon." I'd become so accustomed to the question of "When are you due?" being followed with "How old is your first?" that I simply answered, "They'll be twenty months apart" to virtually any question. ("Room for cream?" they'd ask. "Twenty months!" I'd shout.)

Though I'd never been the source of an angry pregnant woman's rant before, I was familiar with the rhetoric. I'd heard from mothers with one child tired of being asked when they're having another, bottle-feeding parents being lectured by strangers about how "breast is best," and pregnant women so worn down by their bellies being fondled by strangers that they print up T-shirts with the message, "You can touch my belly if I can punch your face."

And truly, I sympathize with how annoying it is to repeat things. Long before I wanted to tattoo "twenty months apart" on my forehead, I worked in the service industry, including at a Starbucks without a bathroom. I know! An abomination. Can you imagine how many times I said, "I'm sorry. We don't have a restroom, but there are facilities at the Rite-Aid and Denny's." (Also, several times to the managers of Rite-Aid and Denny's: "I would *never* imply that our customers should use your bathroom!")

I do not mind being asked if it is hard having kids so close in age. I don't even mind if people ask if they're twins, and it's no problem if they hint around at asking if my birth spacing was intentional. The answer is no, their spacing was not intentional, but it was hard to get and stay pregnant with my first so I hoped that my second would come by surprise and boy, did he. I dare not complain about him arriving so quickly on the heels of his big sister because I am grateful to have him. And yes, having two-under-two's was hard. That shit is no joke.

I don't mind the curiosity of strangers because I am curious about strangers. If I ask a mom if she wants more kids, there is no right answer in my mind. I'm making conversation. If she's uncomfortable with the question, she can decline to answer. She doesn't have to take to her blog to passive aggressively lambast that nosey mom she met at the park. I am not sure where the line is between making small talk and prying, so I make guesses and hope I don't piss people off too much. It's okay when people decline to answer my questions or ask me something that I don't want to answer. I know there are numbskulls out there who lecture parents about how only children are deprived without siblings, but let's not confuse them with normal people who unknowingly ask a question that treads on a recent miscarriage. Making small talk in a diverse society is difficult. Based on the tone of many mommy blogs, we all should immediately cease having any public conversations about having children or being parents, but that's a bit antisocial, no?

Hormonal pregnant women ought to know that some people are in awe of the idea of a human swimming inside another. Not everyone is "judging" anything. These days, we are raising our children in relative isolation, no longer bolstered by large extended families and neighbors bearing casseroles to mark life's big events, and many of us don't have family or friends who will hear out our questions. I had kids while still in my twenties in Los Angeles, where most career-oriented women don't start peeing on the stick until they're in their mid-thirties. Short on friends going through similar experiences, I relied upon strangers for information about where the best playgrounds were and how I was supposed to know when my baby was ready for a sippy cup. In the process, I have certainly asked an impertinent question or two (or ten or twenty) and I remembered that when someone asked me something like, "Is that normal behavior?" when my then two-year-old was rolling around under the table at a restaurant, willing only to eat food passed down to him as if he were a pet dog. (My answer: "Yes, toddlers can be idiosyncratic.") Parents are so accustomed to fending off the unsolicited judgment of strangers that we don't know how to recognize when someone is just trying to talk to us. I hope that none of those more experienced parents mistook my ignorance for judgment, and I try to do the same for all the strangers I meet.

But I didn't know how to respond to the pregnant woman's lecture in the yoga studio, just as I didn't know what to say when a friend, the mother of an adopted son of a different race than her own, complained to me about people asking where he came from. She begrudged the nosiness of strangers and, like the mother-of-twins-to-be, the way their questions were implicitly prying into matters she thought were between her and her doctors. When strangers asked if her son was adopted, she, still raw from years of invasive treatments and heartbreak, felt that what they were really saying was, "So, you couldn't make your own baby?"

Those people probably suspected that there was an interesting story behind my friend and her son. Indeed, there was a story, one about surgeries on polycystic ovaries, a college freshman who hid her pregnancy until the very end and then chose to give the baby up, a story of desperation and love. That's what people wanted to hear, though my friend couldn't reasonably be expected to recount four years of obstacles and miracles for every stranger in the park. She's not obligated to explain her family to everyone, but some of us are simply trying to be social at the playground and maybe learn a little from the people around us.

Pregnant women and babies are captivating because they tell a part of a story, or different parts of different stories: the end of struggle with infertility, the beginning of a new biography, the middle of a transition from woman to woman/mom. Privacy and community are fundamentally at odds, and it's understandable that many parents, including the pregnant mom of twins I offended at the yoga studio, would rather stick with the people they know.

However, I urge the moms-to-be of the world to not print up their hostility towards strangers on a maternity T-shirt and maybe knock it off with the "Shit People Say to Pregnant Women" videos on YouTube and blog posts about the same. I will never argue that people aren't obnoxious—I mean, hell, I'm one of the more obnoxious ones!—but when people shut down conversations before they start or ridicule strangers for not knowing any better, they make themselves difficult to befriend, comfort, console, or support. We all have the option of responding to lame comments in different ways: be funny, charge right back at them, or avoid the conversation.

I was quite bristly throughout my pregnancy with my first child, mostly because it was my fourth pregnancy after three miscarriages. I didn't like acknowledging my pregnancy because I was terrified that it wouldn't yield a baby and I would let strangers down, irrational though it may be. My feeling was, "No one look at me or make me talk about this and then we'll make up for lost time if this all turns out okay." But one day, well into my third trimester, a woman very kindly asked if she could give my belly a pat and I said she could. As she gingerly put her hand on my tummy, she said, "I've never been able to have kids so I think it's so nice when a pregnant woman lets me feel the baby. I've always wondered what it's like to be pregnant." And though I thought being "with child" was excruciatingly difficult in every way, I was so happy to be able to be so. Being pregnant is fucking torture (I get nauseous just thinking about it—daily I suppress an urge to run up to all pregnant women saying, "Oh, no! I'm sorry. Can I get you some tea and a foot massage?"), but being pregnant is a privilege. Likewise, being the partner of a pregnant lady is (possibly even more of) a privilege, or being the parent of any creature who results from a pregnancy is a privilege, an unambiguously wonderful privilege. And that is why one should never crap on the awe of strangers.

It's a hard thing to keep in mind when some random person wants the kind of access to your body that you previously restricted to your partner and obstetrician. But be nice. Understand that being one person with multiple heartbeats inspires deference. Try to enjoy the attention no matter how complicated the feelings it brings up are and remember that potential gropers can be deterred with polite words, not an overly aggressive T-shirt, a lecture, or a series of YouTube videos.

THE BIRTH OF NOBLE SAVAGE FEVER

Knowing that my second child was going to be my last, I wanted his birth to be *perfect;* nothing short of a spiritual awakening. Like, if I had my way, it was going to be a bonanza of exaltation in the delivery room.

My first delivery was totally fine: healthy mother, healthy baby. However, she had come early, suddenly, and quickly. I had meant to forego an epidural, but once my water broke and I was bowled over with pain, I gave in. As the anesthesiologist was inserting the epidural, I wailed through contractions, leading him to pithily remark, "And you're only a centimeter dilated?" I felt like a huge sissy at the time. However, I later realized that I must have been in transition when he was putting in the epidural. My daughter was born less than an hour later. So I guess I could have made it without pain meds—neither my doctor nor I realized how quickly labor was progressing. No matter. It all turned out fine.

I didn't feel bad about having the epidural, but it did gnaw at me a bit when I heard the home birthers amongst my friends describe how accomplished they felt to deliver "naturally"; how amazing the experience was; how totally liberated they felt by their birth choices. When I was pregnant again—and for the last time—I was resolute that I would have a natural birth. However, what I meant when I said "natural" was "spiritually awakening" (whatever that means), though I never would have admitted it.

Women are extraordinarily lucky for all the choices we get to make when it comes to childbirth. However, choices come with a cost, and that cost is ambivalence, competitiveness, and perfectionism; all of which plagued me in the weeks before my son was born. I didn't need Ricki Lake and *The Business of Being Born* to tell me that the Caesarian section rate in the United States is unnaturally and dangerously high, nor did I lose sight of the fact that C-sections, when utilized responsibly, are an incredible life-saving procedure for mothers and babies alike.

As long as my baby wasn't breach or otherwise complicated, I was all but guaranteed a quick labor, and because of that luxury, I became obnoxiously fussy about my birth options. I researched home births, but midwives weren't covered by my insurance and the out-of-pocket cost was huge. Plus, if I arranged a home birth but ended up needing a hospital birth (as I would if I went into labor before thirty-seven weeks—something likely to happen since my first was born at thirty-six-and-a-half weeks), I would have to pay for two births. Instead, I hired a doula, talked to my incredibly patient doctor about how I didn't want an epidural, and then dreamed of how transformed I would be by bravely foregoing pain meds. I wanted this birth to be more than just a bodily function.

I spent a lot of time on natural birth websites and found that the movement's tenets—basically, that medical interventions should be minimized if possible—are nearly universally agreed upon, but some of its followers have misunderstood that idea to mean that *all* interventions are unnecessary. As is often the way in parenting controversies, the people with the most extreme views tend to be the loudest, and so natural birth message boards are crawling with people stricken with an affliction that I call Noble Savage Fever, which is a tendency to romanticize pre- or nonindustrial societies as somehow more pure than our "civilized" one. That is some ignorant crap. For starters, it's based upon a reductionist idea of what nonindustrial life looks like, often by people who think Africa is a country.

Those stricken with Noble Savage Fever show up in a variety of parenting controversies. They're the ones who argue that, since breastfeeding was the preindustrial norm, formula is immoral, though they rarely realize that co-nursing and wet nursing were also norms and that baby feeding vessels show up in the archaeological record as early as 2000 BC. But the fever burns brightest amongst birth extremists.

Okay, ladies with Noble Savage Fever. You want to mother like hunter-gatherers? Okay, let's say you're a !Kung woman living in the Kalahari Desert in the latter part of the twentieth century. Not long after you get your period (probably when you're about sixteen), a dude in his twenties or thereabouts will be shipped over from another tribe, and you'll become betrothed. You do not choose your husband as love marriages aren't a thing there, which is one reason why *When Harry Met Sally* has never been translated into !Kung. You'll give birth by yourself in the bush and then walk back to the village with your newborn. That is unless there is a critical shortage of food at the time of the birth, because then, welp, you might not be welcome to take your baby back to the village. But if you do take home a healthy child, you'll breastfeed for three to five years, and if you don't make enough milk then other nursing women will help. Then you get to raise your children with the help of many villagers and it's all pretty groovy from there. Er, except for the part where you'll have on average four or five kids, two or three of whom may die in infancy or childhood.

Say you want to make the case for "natural" parenting. You're going to leave out the occasional instances of infanticide, which is fine because it doesn't come up that often and even less so in recent decades. But then you're going to leave off the part about co-nursing because to most Americans that idea is icky, even if it is a normal practice in many parts of the world and at many points in human history. Instead, lactivists continue to beat the drum that every woman is able to nurse, despite the numerous women who can't (evident both in the historical and prehistorical record, and in modern practice, but more on that later). And certainly you're going to overlook the arranged marriage thing because of our cultural obsession with love and romance. You might even gloss over the unassisted childbirth. So, instead, you'll focus on the collectivist attitudes towards raising children (i.e. "it takes a village") and the laid-back take on sexuality and childbirth. But cherry picking from cultural traditions without acknowledging—or even understanding—the larger context is problematic. All of this fashionable primativism is bourgeois bullshit, like wearing a Navajo-print thong from Urban Outfitters, except with a child's life at stake.

I am not a hunter-gatherer and neither are you, so stop it. Welcome to the twenty-first century in the industrialized world! Isn't it neat that maternal and infant deaths during childbirth are so rare? And that even extraordinarily fragile premature newborns can go on to thrive? That we can repair complications of childbirth like rectovaginal fistulae, and women in the industrialized world don't have to walk around leaking feces out of their vaginas for the rest of their lives? It is idiotic to idolize indigenous people for their perceived purity, or fail to understand that non-industrial life comes with a heightened risk of childhood disease and injury during childbirth. We have access to incredible technologies that yes, are sometimes wielded in clumsy or downright oppressive ways, but that does not mean that they shouldn't be used when necessary. We need to change the misuse, not stop using them.

Non-industrial life can come with resource instability that's much more daunting than not being able to pay a cable bill. Most of these people who are into "going native" have never been thirsty and not had access to drinking water, and no, the time they went hiking and forgot their Nalgene bottle doesn't count. Nor does that time when they had to work late, and there was nothing in the vending machines but Funyuns give them any understanding of famine. Distaste for the mania of the Western world is not the same as becoming simpatico with a cardboard cutout of a brown woman nursing in a hut. Sure, have a healthy wariness towards the medical establishment, but do not use non- and pre-industrial women to argue against the value of medicine.

And don't even get me started on the Paleo Diet.

The natural birth movement is mostly populated by sane and wise women reacting to real problems in medical culture, particularly an egregious overuse of interventions. But I am going to lose my shit if the Noble Savage Fever brigade keeps trotting out "all of human history" to justify eschewing the entirety of the medical establishment. In an interview, the formerly hat-obsessed sitcom actress/natural parenting advocate, Mayim Bialik, said, "There are those among us who believe that if the baby can't survive a home labor, it is okay for it to pass peacefully. I do not subscribe to this, but I know that some feel that . . . if a baby cannot make it through birth, it is not favored evolutionarily." It's *just super* that Bialik doesn't subscribe to letting babies die to defend some hackneyed ideal of "evolution," but the fact that there are those who do is a problem. Bialik could afford to be a little more concerned with the fact that she's gallivanting around with people who are content to let children die to prove a point about some distorted idea of "natural."

That said, home births can be a fantastic option for some mothers, but not everyone. Midwives are expensive. Many areas don't have birthing centers. And lots of people have risk factors that make hospital deliveries the safest option. But mothers *can* have a good hospital birth. Doctors aren't all out to oppress women. Moms can go into the hospital armed with intelligence and knowledge. They can decline interventions that they believe are unnecessary—as long as we're all clear on the fact that obstetricians attend hundreds, if not thousands of births, and know a few things that a first-time birthing mother might not. If mothers want, they can bring a doula to the hospital who will advocate for their needs and provide more customized support. Partners can be pre-programed with caveats like, "No matter what, don't let me get an epidural" or "No matter what, make sure they get that epidural in me" or "No matter what, don't eat a cheeseburger in front of me if I'm not allowed to partake." (That last one comes from experience.)

Here's my three-point plan for having the best birth for you: 1) Find a doctor or midwife who is awesome; 2) Be assertive; 3) Know that a little deference might be required.

I know birth plans are popular—I know because I made one during my fanatical attempt to have a "spiritual" birth—but they're not the best tactic when dealing with something as unpredictable as childbirth. It's a fine exercise to do on your own and discuss with your doctor, but maybe leave the printout at home on the big day? No doctor wants typed instructions from an amateur.

Though childbirth comes with some risks, we live in an era in which maternal and infant injury and death rates are supremely low, even if some of that is the result of a medical culture that has disenfranchised birthing mothers for a few generations. Yes, there is a birthing-industrial complex, but within that complex are many doctors, midwives, and nurses who want moms to have a good birth experience and a healthy baby. And this is key: Just because C-sections are overused, it doesn't mean that *you* don't need one.

After much hand-wringing about having the perfect birth, I finally went into the delivery room. I had been walking around for weeks five centimeters dilated, which, true story, sucked really hard and was super painful. I begged for an induction, which was goofy because my doctor offered it, and he really didn't need me to sob in his chair and plead, "Get this baby out of me. Can't you see I'm suffering?" It was really unneeded and a little melodramatic. I apologized later.

Here's my birth story: My doctor broke my water at ten thirty in the morning, gave me Pitocin at eleven, and my son was born at one in the afternoon. Not gonna lie, it wasn't the best two and a half hours of my life, but it was fine. I didn't have an epidural because this time the doctor had wised up to how quickly I can pop them out, and it turned out to be a really similar experience to my first delivery. The epidural made very little difference. I'm sure pain meds are fantastic for women in long labors who need to rest before pushing, or for whatever reason anyone wants one, but in my experience giving birth was the same with and without: it hurt, then it hurt more, and then it hurt less. Being free of pain meds didn't cause me to hallucinate that I was a sprouting tree, or make me able to smell harmony. It happened how it happened and I didn't really have all that much control, which is basically what the majority of natural birthers say: If you step out of the way, childbirth happens. And so it did, undramatically, but wonderfully. It was not a spiritual experience, but it was a good one. I have no complaints and I realize how fortunate that makes me.

I had two easy births, something I attribute to Maupin's Rule. In *Tales of the City*, Amisted Maupin wrote that in San Francisco it is impossible to have a good job, a good apartment, and a good man at the same time. (Carrie Bradshaw said the same of New York City in *Sex and the City*, but Maupin came first.) Maupin's Rule applies to pregnancy, childbirth, and the first three months of babies' lives when they're still gummy fetuses blinking back the light, which is sometimes called the fourth trimester. A Facebook poll of my friends (so science, basically) proves this. Rarely, someone struggles with all three, but no one gets off the hook entirely, at least not with their first baby. It even applies to adoptive parents— they might get to skip the pregnancy and childbirth stuff and even sometimes the new baby stuff, but instead they get slammed with bureaucracy, paper work, and a myriad of other complications. Having kids by any means is never easy. In my case, I paid for my easy births by being totally incapacitated during the last few months of pregnancy. I would have a thousand more births, care for a thousand more newborns, but under no circumstances will I ever be pregnant again. It is *the worst*. Or so says me. I'm not in the majority on that one.

I don't doubt that delivery is a spiritually intense experience for some women, but for me it was the first day that I got to hang out with a new kid, which is no small thing. It would be silly to begrudge my easy, uncomplicated births for not being more soul shattering. I'm crazy-grateful for my kids and the easy labors that preceded their healthy deliveries. Maybe if I'd done it in a kiddie pool it would have been more profound? It doesn't matter. Childbirth is (usually) just one shitty day that (usually) ends as a really great day. I wish I could go back in time and stop myself from obsessing over "my" labor (phrased as if I were the one being born) as something more than getting a baby out of my body and into his family's arms. I've received the mom script and know that I'm supposed to say that the days my children were born were the best days of my life, but that would be a lie. It's like saying the best day of a vacation was arriving, not that raising children should ever be compared to a vacation. Yes, the experience of birth matters and mom is a huge player in that, but ultimately it's about the baby, about adding someone new to the world, and beginning a lifelong relationship.

THEY DON'T COME WITH INSTRUCTION MANUALS FOR A REASON

P arents have a reputation for being obnoxious, and not for nothing. I was once not a parent and I recall how annoying I thought it was when people jabbered about milestones and bragged about a kid rolling over like it was somehow an actual accomplishment. I was once bored by people's videos of a baby doing nothing and regular updates about weight gained since the last checkup. Of course, now that I'm a parent, that stuff is basically mom porn and I understand how thrilling that first roll really is, but I get why people other than the parents and grandparents of small children tune out.

The gist of all those updates, however, is that the parents are really excited about what their baby is doing; they're engaged in their baby's world, and even if the obsession is a bit unbecoming, it's a reflection of love and devotion. A new parent who won't stop talking about how their baby breastfeeds like a pro is a person who is really excited to be a parent, and that's to be commended, not shunned.

However, there's another breed of parent jabber that's noxious. We all think our baby is the best in the world, but most of us also know that every other parent thinks the same thing. Some parents seem to think that they really are winning at parenthood, and those people are assholes. The people who think this way are a small minority of parents, and they were probably assholes before they had kids, so really it's a continuation of a character flaw, not a mind state created by becoming a parent.

Not surprisingly, it turns out that a lot of these people populate message boards and blogs, possibly because they can't make friends in real life. Some of these folks truly believe that they're doing everything right and thus it's merely a public service when they take to their blogs to announce, "If you're not attachment parenting, then you're not really parenting." These are the people who sit at their computers and pronounce, "Anyone who doesn't use cloth diapers is an enemy of the environment," or "If you breastfeed in public, you're just lazy and gross." This variety of parenting commentator runs the gamut from conservative Christian disciplinarians to eco-warriors/vegans/homesteaders but all are way too certain about what is best for other people.

Some of this type of web content is really popular, I think perhaps because some people like to be told what to do with utter surety. However, the only thing I'm sure of is that one must never be too sure. Take Janet Lansbury, a former actress and model married to Angela Lansbury's nephew, now a parenting guru espousing the Resources for Infant Education (R.I.E.) method developed by Magda Gerber. The main idea of R.I.E. (pronounced "wry") is that infants should be respected as humans from the outset. It's not an objectionable idea, but as with all parenting methods, there are rules and set guidelines of what is right and wrong in parenting, chiefly that except when meeting their diapering, feeding, bathing, and sleeping needs, babies should be left alone in order to foster independence.

Compare and contrast with the Sears family of doctors, headed up by Dr. William Sears, who advocate for attachment parenting (A.P.), which is almost the same as R.I.E. except that it's the complete opposite. The Sears believe that babies should be held as often as possible (ideally by "wearing" them) and emphasize bonding by breastfeeding and togetherness.

Many parents combine these seemingly contradictory methods—which makes lots of sense, actually. A loose interpretation of both methods combined can be a good fit for a lot of babies and parents. I had one baby who always wanted to be held (à la A.P.) and one who wanted the freedom to explore independently (à la R.I.E.). Both methods have lots of good ideas and tips for dealing with newborns. However, neither method alone is the best practice for all babies and it's utter foolishness that Janet Lansbury and the Sears family continue to preach to parents about what they think is the One True Way to parent a newborn. Babies are all different and parents must be adaptable. Both R.I.E. and A.P. are alluring because they purport to have all the answers, but no one system has all the answers about all babies. Janet Lansbury and the Sears family offer useful advice and provide a great service to parents, yet they often cross over into putting undue stress on parents by guilt tripping working mothers (Sears) or—by far the most bizarre tenant of R.I.E.— insisting that parents ask an infant's permission before they pick the child up.

However, Janet Lansbury (and by extension Magna Gerber) and the Sears family aren't the worst out there. The worst are their disciples, the many bloggers who parrot their teachings and are often less restrained and responsible than the more polished experts. It's tempting to think that after reading some of Magda Gerber's and Dr. William Sears's books that one can become an expert on parenting and is thus qualified to offer advice to every other parent out there. I don't have a firm opinion on the tenants of A.P.—it is clearly a useful model for some people—but I do have a very certain opinion about A.P. message boards and blogs: they suck. They are full of one-upmanship, fruitless comparisons, and competitiveness. No one is the most attachment-y attachment parent out there, so everyone can stop trying.

I have similar ire for the occasional practice of including signatures listing one's parenting credentials. Early in my time as a mother, I subscribed to a listserv for local parents and—hand to God—there was a woman with the following signature: "BFing, BWing, and AP MAMA to 2 yr old," which translates to "breast-feeding, baby-wearing, and attachment parenting mama to a two-year-old," and then she listed the poor kid's name and birthday. That right there is a vomit sundae. How right does a person have to think she is to list all of her parenting practices in her damn signature? If I still participated in message boards, my signature would be, "My kids are fine."

This same woman wrote, "There is nothing more magical than practicing A.P. The bond we have with him and with each other is so intimately connected and so intensely strong. It is true spiritual nourishment and love that we give each other in being an A.P. family." There is nothing more wonderful and banal than the love that a family has for one another, but it is the height of idiocy to think that one family's love is somehow grander than another family's because of a particular parenting practice. Parents managed to love their children before Dr. Sears came around. Likewise, parents figured out how to put their babies down and get some shit done around the house before Magna Gerber told them it might be beneficial to do so.

I wholly sympathize with the urge to find a parenting manual and stick to it because, of course, I'm a gigantic hypocrite. When my first was born, I tried hard to be a good attachment parent and followed all the rules. I didn't know what else to do. My own parents raised me well, but I wasn't interested in emulating their methods wholesale. I remembered how scared I was sleeping in my own room and how as a small child I longed for more closeness. I wanted that snuggly loveliness for my kids.

Eventually, I figured out how to cultivate all that bonding without following a rulebook. It took a while for me to grow confident in my own skills and instincts as a mother to forego parenting manuals entirely, but I got there. I ended up doing some stuff that fit in well with R.I.E., some stuff that qualifies as A.P., and some stuff that was just my own way of being myself as a mother, which was really the hardest thing for me to learn. And I'd like to say that I learned it in some wonderful way that could be translated into a little story I'd recount here, but the truth is that I learned it by watching some other moms and deciding that I didn't want to be like them.

That's not very nice, I realize. But here's the thing: The gist of attachment parenting is going with baby's flow. And yet, so many attachment parents are super-duper uptight about their attachment parenting and scrupulously maintain nap schedules and rigidly apply the tenets of A.P. whether their baby is into it or not (because remember, some babies hate being held all day). Being that I'm human and thus judgmental, I thought, "Geesh, why don't those parents drop the A.P. manual and parent like themselves and stop pretending that they're going with the flow when clearly, they're not 'going with the flow'—type people?"

As a new parent, I worked very hard to comply with the parent scripts that I had picked up somewhat inadvertently from new mom groups, message boards, listservs, and books. I was working really hard to fit into the model of what a mother should be, rather than being myself. Being a parent isn't like being an account executive or a programmer. It's not a job or a workplace into which one must fit. It's a relationship. My children don't have A Mother. They have me. They have a mom who gets pissed off when people don't use their blinkers when making unprotected left turns and sometimes shouts obscenities in the car. They have a mom who likes to pretend to be Gollum and run around the house growling, "Where are my sneaky little hobbitses? We wants our preciouses!" They have a mom who can't cook, eats ice cream out of the carton, and likes to celebrate October by re-watching every "Treehouse of Horror" episode of *The Simpsons*. They have a mom who will make them listen to short, but highly informative, lectures on primatology during zoo visits and a mom who is passionate about a few things *other* than them. I convey love and trust for my children by asking them to accept me for who I am and I offer them the same in return.

When they were born, I didn't start a new "job"; we began a relationship. I bond with them by letting them get to know me, hacky Gollum impersonation and all. They don't have a perfect mom, but they have a mom who loves them perfectly, and that's what is not covered in parenting manuals. That's why swaddling versus co-sleeping versus bottle-feeding versus cloth-diapering versus scheduled naps doesn't really matter.

Listen to how adults talk about their own parents. When I whine that I wish my parents had been more snuggly with me when I was little, I'm not talking about co-sleeping. I'm talking about an ineffable vibe that was not the result of any particular parenting practice. They could have co-slept with me because a manual told them to, but the feeling would not have changed. And likewise, when I reminisce about the relative freedom I had as a child, say being able to walk to the library by myself, I'm chipper about it because I didn't feel abandoned, I felt trusted. Again, the quality of my memories is traced to some nebulous feeling I had, not the actual practice. It's not what a parent does that matters (well, give or take a little), but all the woogly-googly, difficult-to-describe moods, vibes, and feelings surrounding it. No adult is ever going to say, "Thanks, Mom and Dad, for following Dr. Sears's tenets to a T, because all that structured bonding made me a well-adjusted adult," or "Thank goodness you read all of Magda Gerber's books because now I have a true sense of independence and confidence in myself." Growing up is too multifaceted and complicated to pin on infant care, so long as parents truly love and provide for their children with the best of intentions. It's not the methods that matter, it's the parent. Gurus have their uses, but in the end, parenting isn't work that can be optimized. It's much fuzzier and more individualized than that.

So, this one time, I wrote a little article for the *Huffington Post* and my life became a non-stop morass of nonsense. Good times . . .

In the article, I "came out" as pro-vaccine. I talked a bit about Jack and Clio, two children who I know through their moms' blogs. Because the universe is viciously unfair, Jack and Clio have leukemia. Due to the treatment they must undergo, they are unable to be given some vaccines. Those two particular children had their shots when they were younger and probably still have some immunity, but vaccines are not 100 percent effective and if they were exposed to, say, measles, it could make them very ill and be an arduous complication in their treatment. Jack and Clio are two very good reasons for why every single able-bodied child should receive vaccines. They couldn't be protected from leukemia, but they can be protected from chickenpox, and thus it is the responsibility of all parents to be freaking decent human beings and vaccinate their kids to protect them as well as other individuals.

You know who else is vulnerable? Babies. Itty-bitty babies who can't get vaccines. Also, pregnant women. Also, immuno-compromised individuals of all ages including very young children with lifelong illnesses, and adults with HIV or a variety of other chronic illnesses. Also, old people. The entire point of bothering to organize ourselves into something resembling a society is to protect those people.

The anti-vaccine movement is different from every other parenting-related controversy in that it is measurably dangerous, and not only for unvaccinated children, but for lots of other folks. I might not believe much in colloidal silver or other alternative medicines that haven't been proven to work, and I don't care what anybody does with that stuff. But I care if people aren't vaccinating their kids. It's not just a personal choice or an individual's private business. An unvaccinated child who picks up pertussis might be okay once the cough subsides, but in the meantime the choices of that child's parents could have inadvertently killed a newborn.

Since publishing that article, I have spent a great deal of time interacting with people who range from vaccine denialists to those who are merely vaccine-hesitant—which is not such a terrible thing to be, as long as one appropriately weighs the conjecture of a random website against the strength of the conclusions of nearly the entire medical establishment and almost all of the world's governments. As a result, I'm cranky about vaccines, mostly because I can't fathom why we have to defend them at all. The evidence in favor of vaccines is so overwhelming that to continue to oppose them after examining the evidence is dunderheaded at best and evil at worst.

Gather 'round ye folks, for Auntie JJ is going to tell you a tale.

A long time ago, in a galaxy far, far away, there was a woman who lived in a small hamlet on the outskirts of nowhere on a dry planet that we'll call Tatooine because I'm excellent at world creation and I just made that name up from scratch. Let's say there were no books on her planet. Certainly, there was no Internet. There was nothing on this planet except for yurts, crops, and sand (and one bar, but it was a wretched hive of scum and villainy so nice ladies like the one in our story never went there). One day, during a particularly impressive dual sunset—again, I just made up the possibility that there could be a planet orbiting a binary star-based system, totally spawned from my own vivid imagination, as I am that great at world creation—the lady had sex for the first and only time. Nine months later, she had a baby and she knew one thing for sure: Having sex during an arousing double sunset is how babies are made.

Before the next dual sunset, she went to every yurt she could find and informed the villagers, "If you have sex now, you'll have a baby!" Some of the villagers were like, "Huh. We had five kids, maybe all of them were conceived during a dual sunset and we didn't realize it." Another responded, "Yes, that must be it! Because though we have sex, we have never conceived the children we wanted. It must be because we haven't had sex during the dual sunset!" And another said, "Now we know to never have sex during the gorgeous double sunset and we can be certain to remain childless so we can save up to buy a bitchin' new XP-38 landspeeder."

And that right there is how an anecdote can mix with confirmation bias to create an old wives' tale. The family that wanted babies might have been lucky and ended up with a pregnancy shortly thereafter, and the family that didn't want to conceive might have ended up never conceiving. That lady would have looked like a genius! Or, more likely, her suspected correlation might have ended up being randomly true some of the time and wrong most of the time, but remained as a myth because, as my obstetrician explains it, when people are certain of their baby's sex before birth, they're right half the time and the rest of the time they actually knew deep down that they were wrong.

But let's look at another version of my tale:

A long time ago, in a galaxy far, far away, there was a woman on Tatooine who was curious about how the universe worked and where babies came from, specifically if there was any link between sex during an arousing double sunset and conception. She developed a study plan and asked all of her fellow villagers to create logs of when they had sex and when they gave birth and then she examined the data to see if it was more likely for babies to be conceived after sex during a period when the two suns of the system set within a few minutes of each other or within whatever unit of time these fine folks, or perhaps a republic of neighboring galaxies, had established as a metric, given that every planet most likely orbits their respective heat and light source at different speeds. (Gee, this world creation stuff gets complicated.) In order to get a large enough data set, she, um . . . tracked it for many generations? Or, er, traveled to many villages and asked residents to keep logs as well. In any case, she came up with a substantial enough quantity of data to do a decent analysis and discovered that the suns had nothing to do with conception. And hey, maybe she also figured out the pattern of ovulation and pioneered fertility counseling for all the denizens of Tatooine.

These two stories are the difference between anecdotal evidence and actual evidence. I'll let you guess which one is prevalent amongst people who do not vaccinate.

But science is the antidote to anecdotes. It's not a real debate: Vaccinate your children. Vaccinate them on schedule and according to your doctor's suggestions. If you want to delay one or more vaccines, discuss the risks and benefits with your doctor. And dear sweet humanity, I cannot underline this enough: *Talk to an actual doctor, and no, Dr. Google does not count.*

Let's pretend you "don't believe" in vaccinating your kid so you can join me over here for a chat about the vaccine non-debate/debate.

"But, JJ," you might say. "I did my research." Stop it. No you didn't. I know me some science. I've taken lots of college-level science courses. I understand vaccinology a little bit, but ultimately I don't know anything. Why? I'm not a goddamned doctor! Listen to your doctor! Not the Internet!

I didn't go to medical school and neither did you (unless you did, then props). You and me both—we have massive gaps in our knowledge. Reading a few Wikipedia entries does not make one an authority. Because not all of us can fathom the intricacies of medicine, we rely on trained professionals to do that for us: doctors, nurses, nurse practitioners, research physicians, etc. And I'm talking about real medical professionals, not the fame-whoring purveyors of bullshit who sometimes have TV shows, and certainly not Dr. Jay Gordon, pediatrician to superstar vaccine denialists Mayim Bialik and Jenny McCarthy.

"Oh," you say, "well too bad for you because I really have done the research." Again, no you did not. The research is not subjective and the consensus of existing research is that vaccines are safe and valuable. I've now spent a truly grotesque amount of time engaging with the anti-vaccine movement. While I am not an expert on vaccines, I am an expert on anti-vaxxers, and one thing I know for certain is that they are nearly uniformly ignorant and do not understand how to interpret research. That said, there are a few vaccine denialists with enough scientific skills to twist existing research to appear to support their imagined conclusions.

"You're just a shill for big pharma," they'll say. Stop it! How does one even become a shill for big pharma? At this point, I *should* be a shill for big pharma. Where my big pharma goodies at? Merck! Hop to it! But what does this charge even mean? It's obviously in the best financial interest of drug companies for there to be tons of sick people, which is what would happen if everyone stopped vaccinating. Think of all of the potential prescriptions! Furthermore, it seems that those who profit most off of the vaccine debate/non-debate are the denialists. Take Dr. Jay Gordon. He sells 105-minute multi-chapter streaming webinars on his website, has created a DVD titled *Vaccinations?*—seriously, with a question mark—and a book, *Preventing Autism: What You Can Do to Protect Your Children Before and After Birth*. Let's not dwell on the fact that there's no proven way to "protect" children from autism nor the troubling ramifications of suggesting that it's something from which children need to be protected, because, well, we'll get to that.

But suppose you insist on denying that vaccines are beneficial for everyone and you say, "Lay off me. It's a personal choice." A lot of things are choices. Technically, I could personally *choose* to stand in the middle of a shopping mall with a machete in each hand and swing my arms willy-nilly, but then I'd be choosing to commit a crime and endanger my fellow shoppers. So yeah, I guess you technically have the choice to endanger immuno-compromised individuals and other vulnerable members of the community, but it's a bad choice. If you make that choice, then you are wrong.

The article I wrote for the *Huffington Post* reflected a much calmer attitude than I have now. However, because it went "viral" (and hang on for a second while I restrain myself from making an all too obvious pun . . . okay; we're good now), that article was read by potentially millions of people and thus caused my life to become a mess of vaccine-related emails, messages, tweets, and comments. As a result, I learned that the anti-vaccine movement is even more vicious and ignorant than I had ever understood. They often resorted to insulting me personally and spewed nonsense easily contradicted by citing peer-reviewed science, but refused to change their course despite overwhelming evidence of their wrongness.

When writing about parenting, wrongness is a tricky notion. After all, as Dr. Jay Gordon says, "No one knows your child better than you do." And it's true. My husband and I know our kids better than anyone else knows them and we take our responsibility to care for them very seriously. We are deeply connected to our children and, at least for a while longer, we know them better than they know themselves. Oftentimes, I know what my kids are thinking. Like, I can literally read their adorable little minds and anticipate that they're about to stage an attack on the Christmas tree using a stepladder and a fairy wand. And I have all sorts of woobly-woggly instincts and gut feelings about them and constantly adjust the ways I deal with them in response to these difficult-to-define instincts.

So yes, parenting is instinctive and individualized. And thus, the overriding message of a lot of writing about parenting (including sometimes my own) is that each of us are the best equipped to make choices for our own children. And while there is a lot of scolding parenting writing out there (including sometimes my own), what people generally prefer to read are articles about how it's hard for everyone, we're all doing our best, and let's just support one another, m'kay? However, when those ideas are taken to their logical extreme, what we have are a lot of parents who think they understand more than their doctors, indeed more than the entire medical and scientific establishment, and thus they prioritize instinct over reason when, actually, good parenting involves both.

Parents' instincts can misfire. Sometimes we have to protect our children from our worst instincts and, say, talk ourselves out of putting down a screaming baby and walking out of the house, possibly all the way to the Mexican border and starting a new life as a childless Zapatista. Because in a few minutes, that won't be what we want. Those are just emotions getting the best of us because we've been up for five nights in a row nursing a baby through a cold, and we're tired, and why won't this baby stop crying because we can't do any more than we're already doing, and oh my gosh, we have to pee because when was the last time we put this baby down, and are we seriously going to have to sit on the toilet holding the baby because that's a gross and desperate thing to do but that's what our life has become and we read about these rad Zapatista women back when we were in college, and even though they live in the jungle fighting the government (or something, we forget the specifics), their lives are probably a lot better than ours are right now, and whoops, the baby just puked down our shirt, and the spit-up is actually welling up in our nursing bra, and the baby still hasn't stopped crying, and why didn't anyone tell me that this is what parenting is going to be like?

That's the fight or flight instinct kicking in and landing on flight even though fleeing is a very unkind thing to do to a baby. Not that what I described has ever happened to me, but if it did, it got a little better in a few minutes and then a lot better in a few days and I'm really glad I'm not a Zapatista right now. Both fight and flight are two good examples of instinctive urges that should often be ignored when parenting. Certainly at least physical fighting because that's also known as beating your kid and that's not just one of those arbitrary no-no's. It's a fundamental abdication of parental duties.

Parents who don't vaccinate, no matter how much they say they've "done the research," are an example of instincts gone awry, though certainly not to the same degree as in the cases of parents who beat their children, because, let's get real, this is a book, not the Internet, and such superlative insults don't belong here. Parents who don't vaccinate are not an evil conspiracy dead set on endangering newborns. Sometimes parents don't vaccinate to conform to their ultra-crunchy or, conversely, ultra-conservative community, and their urge to have normative values suppresses critical thinking. Sometimes parents don't vaccinate because an alternative medical practitioner (or, in rare cases, a conventional medical practitioner) has given them misinformation.

Pediatricians and other doctors can sometimes be very rushed, and many people have positive experiences seeking medical care outside of the traditional medical establishment. It's a lot easier to swallow the advice of an acupuncturist who has spent hours talking to you than it is a physician who spent five minutes. However, this wouldn't be the first time that compassion and truth are at odds. In the United States, our medical system is not rigged in favor of the individual. There are bad doctors. There are good doctors who are rushed by forces they cannot abate. It's vital to find a doctor who can be trusted and is willing to listen to parents' concerns. There are many obstacles to getting good care, and the overall result is a populace distrustful of the medical establishment. However, the benefits of vaccines have been verified the world over and the conclusions of the vast majority of scientists who have examined this topic should not be dismissed because doctors are sometimes rude.

There are also the parents who operate on a mixture of instinct and Googling: the vaccine hesitant. I understand that vaccines *look* bad. First off, the Internet is riddled with click-baiting, advertising-driven websites so that many of the first websites you encounter when searching for vaccine information are, at best, ignorant, and, at worst, fronts for vitamin and supplement companies. Plus, vaccines seem icky. They often come in syringes, which are what heroin addicts use. Yuck! And they contain gross-seeming stuff like killed or weakened viruses. Ew! And formaldehyde. Barf! And heavy metals. The depravity! Geez, when you look at vaccines like that, they seem downright barbaric. Yet, every ingredient of vaccines has been rigorously studied and tested for safety. Mercury is bound up into thimerosal when added, for safety, though it is rarely even included in vaccines anymore. There's more formaldehyde in an apple than a vaccine. And then, it doesn't help that the pinpricks hurt and often kids have mild vaccine reactions such as fevers or muscle soreness. And it really doesn't help that very, very rarely, children have legitimate adverse reactions that cause lasting damage. However, the risk of a child being damaged by a vaccine is miniscule compared to risk of getting a vaccine-preventable illness.

"No amount of risk is okay with me," you say, because you still insist on denying the obvious benefits of vaccines. "I'm going to take my kid to a chickenpox party so she can get natural immunity." If that's what you're thinking, then let's not mince words: You are a goddamned idiot. Please email me your address and your schedule so that I may come over to your house and personally slap you across the face and confiscate your computer (don't worry, I'll donate it to charity after thoroughly disinfecting it). First of all, are you old enough to have had chickenpox as a child? I am. It was miserable. I wouldn't wish it on my worst enemy—which, incidentally enough, is you, chickenpox party parents—let alone my or anyone else's children. Sure, I survived chickenpox unscathed. Most people who have had it in the last several decades did. However, complications are real and dangerous. An unvaccinated child could infect a pregnant woman or a newborn baby, i.e., folks more likely to have terrible complications. Pregnant women who get it during their first trimester can have babies with low birth weights and defects such as limb abnormalities. Oh, but it's all worth it because you spared your kid one needle prick? Also, have you ever met someone who's had shingles? People who've had chickenpox can sometimes get shingles later in life, and that shit is awful! I watched my grandmother suffer through a bout of it. Of course, there's a shingles vaccine now, but that means nothing to you, I guess.

On the bright side, since publishing that article about vaccines on the *Huffington Post*, I've learned that there aren't actually that many dumdums around who still claim that vaccines cause autism, likely because of the voluminous evidence against that claim. The surgeon and researcher who originally claimed a connection, Andrew

Wakefield, has since been wholly discredited, as his research was fraudulent. Vaccine denialists like to talk about shills for big pharma, but Wakefield was *actually* a shill for big legal. A few families alleged that their children were damaged by the M.M.R. shot. They hired lawyers. The lawyers then paid Wakefield to produce data that would support their claims so that their clients could get big payouts. And thus the tenacious myth that vaccines cause autism was born.

Wakefield's data has never been replicated because it was fabricated. Journalist Brian Deer exposed the money trails. Several studies have since disproven any link between vaccines and autism, including far larger epidemiological studies than the fraudulent one conducted by Wakefield. It was all a big lie and even the most ardent vaccine denialists backed off of it and instead ran with the fact that some vaccines contain mercury. And then, when mercury in vaccines was reduced and/or eliminated, they moved on to aluminum. Though the research supporting the effectiveness of aluminum in vaccines is strong, that's where the bleeding edge of vaccine deniers remain. I'm sure they'll soon move on to something else. Maybe chemicals in the syringes themselves. Maybe the inclusion of animal cells? Who knows! They're a creative lot.

Yet, there are still a few people belaboring the disproven vaccine-autism link. I heard from some parents of autistic children after my article was published. Some of them said, "Thank you," because it is painful for them to have to repeatedly tell strangers that no, they did *not* cause their child's autism by giving them vaccines. Because remember, at its core, the assertion that vaccines cause autism *blames* parents for their child's atypicality. However, there was another group of parents of autistic children who reached out to me to say, "*How dare you!*" They believed that since I did not personally have a child on the spectrum, I could not write about vaccines. This is obviously goofy as there is no relationship between vaccines and autism.

That said, there was one more group of people I came into contact with who impacted me greatly: adults on the autism spectrum. Imagine their experience: It's been repeatedly asserted that their way of being is the result of vaccine *damage*; that they're *damaged*. Even worse, there's a trend amongst parents of young children with autism to work towards a *cure* to heal the *damage*. Imagine how all that looks to an adult with autism or an autism spectrum disorder. Think about the perspective of adults with autism next time Jenny McCarthy opens her damn yap. It all starts to sound even grosser.

Oh, and get your flu shot, too! But don't just take my word for it. Talk to your doctor, and, again, I don't mean Dr. Google.

HOW TO MANAGE BABY'S
SOCIAL CALENDAR

When my daughter was born, one of the many crises I had was due to the fact that I didn't know any other parents of young kids aside from my sisters, who both live far away. I immediately signed up for a nursing support group and joined a local club for mothers. This also helped with one of my other crises: I was bored.

I immediately started filling out my weeks as a stay-at-home mom with new baby playgroups, but what I mean by playgroups is that my baby would flop around on a blanket in front of me while I chatted with other moms who had babies the same age as mine. This was in so many ways constructive. I learned a lot from those other moms. I picked up tricks for breastfeeding discretely in public (wear two shirts—one goes up, one goes down), dealing with diaper rash, and where to get good deals on baby clothes. However, in many other ways, it was corrosive.

Take for example Amy. As happens sometimes, Amy didn't like me. I'd say that it's because she was neurotic, insecure, controlling, and even more obnoxious than me, but I'm sure she would tell it differently. It doesn't matter either way. At one playgroup meeting, Amy went around the circle of babies and listed all the ones who she thought had nice hair, and as expected, skipped over my own cutie face. Now, I'm not just being a proud mama here, but my daughter had, and still has, remarkable hair. She was born with a full head of platinum blonde locks, which I guess is uncommon enough for blonde babies that the nurses at the hospital and the women hosting the nursing support meetings all snapped pics with their cell phones to show people later. I would have loved her as much if she were bald. Platinum blonde hair at birth is not an earned virtue. It's a genetic happenstance. Thus, I do not agree that babies should be ranked into categories of "good hair" and "bad hair."

What stands out in my unbecomingly vivid memory of this incident is not the slight against my daughter, but the question: *Holy hell, why was I spending time with a woman who ranked baby hair?!* Indeed, why was I spending so much time with a woman who disliked me so much? Why did I think that was important?

And because one day a week of playgroups was not enough for me, I joined others and met more people, some of whom were equally as detestable as Amy. Like the woman I will only refer to as Milo Flynne's Mom because that's how she signed her emails. Every time she changed Milo Flynne's cloth diapers, she made a show of it, saying stuff in her cute widdle baby woicey-woice like, "No plastic on your precious baby bottom, Milo Flynne." But the joke isn't on Milo Flynne's Mom. It's on me for hanging around her so much that I grew to despise her. Life is too short to be chummy with people I dislike, no matter how desperate I was for mom friends.

Even with 20/20 hindsight, I can only speculate about my motives for staying in those groups for *over a year*. Part of it was that I liked some of the other mothers enough to welcome their company once a week. I also felt like I owed my baby face time with other babies, even if I was miserable. See, I had this idea that the other babies were my baby's friends, but silly me, babies don't have friends. Even two-year-olds don't really have friends. She wasn't attached to those other babies. I was attached to the idea of her being attached to those other babies.

But the biggest reason that I stayed in that group was that I thought that if I didn't get along with these particular mothers, then I wasn't going to get along with any mothers, so I might as well learn to adapt. This turned out to be untrue. I eventually met some mom friends who I found not only tolerable, but wonderful! They didn't necessarily have kids exactly the same age as mine, but we had other things in common, and that's what really matters. My best mom friends are now also my best friends and we talk about much more than where to get steals on onesies. When I hung with that group at first, what I was really being was impatient. It took time for me to meet these women who I would ultimately bond with about motherhood and womanhood and wifedom and all the other facets of our lives. When my daughter was born, my impulse was to find mom friends instantly, but it took time. I wish that instead of suffering through rankings of baby hair, I had tried harder to find a group that felt genuinely supportive or bonded with individual mothers on a one-on-one basis.

Once my daughter was old enough to be pushed on a swing, I met some fantastic parents and nannies at the playground. An aside: Nannies are truly wonderful people with whom to talk about parenting. Many of them have already raised kids of their own and are fantastically practical and innovative. They know all the good parks, the best shops, and have all the tricks for wrangling kids in the grocery store. Nannies get stuff done and I've learned a lot from them. (Also, in Los Angeles, many of them have worked for famous families and they have some choice celebrity gossip.)

When I started taking my baby to the gym and leaving her in the child care area, I met even more great parents, with whom I sometimes chatted while working out. When my daughter started going to a few mornings of preschool, I met even more great parents. Once I got out in the world in more genuine ways than a weekly arranged "play date" for new babies, the world of parent friends opened up for me. It took time and I only wish I could go back and wait it out instead of trying to force friendships with the mothers who had been randomly assigned to the same playgroup.

Having a new baby is a lot like being a freshman in college. I treated my assigned playgroup like they were my dorm mates, and we were going to stick together through this mom/college thing and forge bonds based on shared experiences. Sure, sometimes people do stay friends with all of unit II, floor eight for the rest of their lives, but most people over the course of freshman year become close with only a handful of people from their dorm because the shared experience of being a freshman at a particular college at a particular time is not enough to build a close relationship. There has to be more of a connection, and finding people with whom a meaningful connection can be forged usually just takes time.

FRESH AIR, GROCERIES, NEW JEANS, AND OTHER THINGS PARENTS NEED

I think of the Internet as a massive starving monster that feeds on page clicks and insecurity. Who's insecure? Teenagers and new parents. Who's all over the Internet generating those page clicks? Teenagers and new parents. And actually, new parenthood is a sort of second adolescence. In the case of pregnant and birthing moms, their entire bodies have changed. Stretch marks may have appeared, boobs have grown, new sweating patterns and smells abound. It's all beautiful, of course. The miracle of new life and all that. But on a fundamental level, it's baffling, gross, and confusing. Just like puberty.

And just as with puberty, there are new responsibilities and new roles. The shift from girl to woman is typically turbulent. Likewise, the shift from woman to mother is fraught with questions, feelings, consternation, and perils. Just as I recall how weird it was to go out in public wearing a bra for the first time, I remember how weird it was to go out in a nursing bra for the first time. Same song, different verse. And in this verse, there's the care and feeding of a brand new human being to attend to.

So no wonder new parents are some of the most insecure creatures on the planet. First, there are the woes pertaining to baby: Is he growing quickly enough? Is it okay that she can only roll over to the right and not to the left? Is his head too flat? And while some solace can be found in groups for new parents, that opens them up to comparing their kid to other people's. Why does Shanae's baby sleep through the night but my baby wakes up constantly? Why can John's kid already hold his neck up but mine still needs support? Both Mark and Marina have babies that like tummy time, but my child acts as if she's being tortured when I put her on her tum! There are probably some chill new parents out there, but I was not one, and I didn't know any.

And I'm guessing whoever those chill new parents are, they don't spend a lot of time on the Internet, because websites and message boards are teeming with parents freaking out about the minutiae of baby's every happening. On one hand, this is healthy and normal. New parents care! They're trying to do what's best! They want their kids to be healthy and normal! But on the other hand, that nonsense can drive a person insane.

Some of the Internet's offerings for new parents are informative and calming. Some of them are cheerily upbeat, about how parents are the most special people in the world and what we do is nothing if not heroic. And some things make new parents even more insecure, like rants about "the lady I saw at the grocery store who let her kid cry while she was in the checkout line instead of taking her baby outside and soothing her." And what is one supposed to take away from that? *I better not be* that *parent.*

Eventually, if one reads enough of those kinds of message boards and articles, it can make one weary about taking a baby out in public. It feeds this idea of *Oh, shit! Everywhere I go with my child, I am being judged,* which is why the Internet has ten bajillion articles about parent judgment. We all become aware that people are examining our parenting wherever we go and this is horribly intimidating. I remember quite acutely suffering through the shift from being an individual who slips into the store to grab a few things to a person with a baby who lumbers through the store with a giant stroller, a squalling kid, and an overflowing diaper bag. It's hard. And then when I realized that not only was I no longer just a person doing her business, but a person who could be the subject of a message board post about new moms who block the aisles with an oversized stroller, or a post about a mom who placated her baby by thrusting snacks at her, or, better yet, a post about those indecent moms who breastfeed while grocery shopping, however discreetly, it all gets to be quite daunting.

Many parents, myself included, deal with a powerful urge to stay home and not deal with nursing in public, or alternatively, getting the side eye from would-be lactivists for bottle feeding. If I stayed home, no one could judge me. No one could be annoyed by my filthy stroller or sometimes noisy infant. No one could think a single damn thought about me, and instead, I could order all my household goods online. Hello, grocery delivery! However, that gets boring and at some point, I had to make a conscious decision to rejoin the outside world with my new sidekick.

I'm not saying this was a graceful process. Once, I took my baby daughter to a Mommy and Me movie and we were running late. I parked, scooped her from her car seat, loaded her in a stroller, and sped off to the movie. When I returned, I found a note on my car scolding me for having touched another person's car with my stroller's rubberized handle, accusing me of scratching her Mercedes. The note was from a woman who was in the next car watching me as I lumbered through the process of loading my kiddo up and *evaluating me*. I hadn't thought much of it while I was dashing off to the movie, although I was embarrassed at being watched, but when I got that note I was furious, and also mortified. There again was a reminder that when I was out with a child, I was always being watched. I was no longer JJ the Woman, but JJ the Mother.

While there are some kind people out there who are excited to see babies and peek in the stroller (and sometimes fondle babies' faces), there are also people out there who believe that babies don't belong in public; that the public sphere is solely for people who are quiet, orderly, and well behaved. This is a problem for parents of babies (and an even bigger problem for parents of toddlers) because just by being a parent in public, some people are angry. However—and this is important—those people are assholes. Babies are tiny little citizens with all the rights of any other person. They're allowed to go to the grocery store. They're allowed to go to the mall. And for goodness sake, they're also allowed to fly on planes.

The existence of these nasty people means that sometimes being in public with a child is an inherently confrontational act, one with which a lot of parents would rather not deal. But new parents need to go shopping too! And sometimes they even need to hop on a plane to introduce baby to Great Grandma Louise because who knows how many Christmases she has left?

Learning to be in public with my baby required me to thicken my skin. Whenever I caught someone examining me with my infant, I stared back. This also worked with public nursing. If someone stared, I stared back until they realized that they were gawking at me. If anyone said something to me like, "Are you sure that your baby is really safe in that carrier?" I answered firmly, "Yes, she's fine." "Are you sure you wouldn't rather go to the restroom to feed her?" "Nope. I'm fine here." "She seems fussy. Shouldn't you feed her?" "Nope. I've got it under control." And I held that stance even when things weren't under control, even when I was a mess, and all I could smell was the spit-up on my shoulder. And then, as a further challenge, I tried to listen when people might have been right. Sometimes it was helpful, like when I'd lost a baby shoe somewhere in the grocery store and because of a stranger's alert, I retraced my steps and was able to find it.

It seems sometimes as if the entire world doubts the competency of new parents, as if we're all constantly in need of supervision, not support, which is frustrating, but there are some genuinely bad parents out there and the public at large doesn't know what kind any given parent is. Perhaps those concerned/judgmental strangers just read a story on the Internet about a baby who died of neglect and they're now worried about all new babies and they're taking it out on every new mom they see.

I had to take my baby out in public because I had to resume being a regular person at some point, and that was something I couldn't do by going out only to attend new parent groups or by interacting with other new parents on the Internet. For the first month or so of my mothering life, I was nothing but JJ the Mother, but eventually I had to also become JJ the Mother and Woman. I needed to not wear maternity jeans for the entire first year of my kid's life, so I went jean shopping . . . with her and she screamed the whole time in the dressing room while I was trying to cram my postpartum ass into normal pants. I missed my favorite restaurants (can we call Chipotle a restaurant?) so I took her with me and breast-fed her discreetly at the table. I longed for a caramel macchiato, so I took her to the coffee shop and struggled to get the door open and pull the stroller through the narrow doorway behind me for the first time.

The time frame for re-entering the world is different for everyone. It may take a year, it may take a day, but it's got to be done at some point. It takes a lot longer for new parents to remember their personality and feel like themselves again, or at least it did for me. It was probably a year before I felt like I had any of my old swagger back (and truthfully, I never fully returned to my old self because the act of caring for a child fundamentally changed me), but the first step was going out in public and faking it. I had to first learn to be in front of strangers, even when that meant fielding comments and looks that ranged from kind to mean-spirited, from undermining to supportive.

I simply couldn't spend any more time on the couch holding my baby and watching reruns of *Wife Swap*. Also, it turned out that my baby was pretty curious about that world and got a kick out of seeing the Mylar balloons in the grocery store and the huge bundles of flowers at the farmer's market. Once I finally got out there, she made it pretty clear that she wanted to see more than her nursery and the inside of my shirt.

SLEEP: NO MATTER WHAT, BABIES PASS OUT EVENTUALLY

Sleep deprivation doesn't hit every parent at the same time. Some parents come home from the hospital bedraggled and don't recover for months, if not years, and some do okay for a while and then get slammed during one growth spurt or another. Some never have any substantial sleep woes, and if that's your experience, let me offer you a piece of advice: *Shhhhh*. No one wants to hear it.

Fortunately, as with most of my sophomore year of college, I've blacked out most of the first six months of my second child's life, because, oy, I was *tired*. I know those months happened—I've seen the pictures—but my memories are spotty at best. If I try to dredge anything up, I get memories like the day all I got to eat were microwaved tamales . . . while standing up . . . while bouncing my fussy baby. I remember comparing my baby to Jack Dorso, Martin Short's character on *Arrested Development*, who despite the loss of use of his lower limbs, insisted on being carried around everywhere by a man he hired named "Dragon." In this scenario I was Dragon and my son hadn't so much lost his mobility as not gained it yet. That baby, he was a shark—always moving, even though he couldn't move. Whenever I think back on it, I start bouncing on my toes and pacing in circles because that is exactly what I did for six months until the wee-beast learned to get himself around.

This constant movement continued through the night, which he regarded as more of a very dark day, and it wasn't enough to hold him or rock him in a chair. The kid needed to move and so I paced the expanse of my cottage all day, and often, all night. That little mofo would just wake right the hell up if I so much as paused to brush my teeth.

It was during this time span that a kindly old woman said to me, "Better enjoy him while he's little." Perhaps it was due to sleep deprivation, but after making this announcement, she began to look to me like one of those giant drumsticks they sell at the Renaissance Faire. I'm happy to say that I have never actually eaten an old woman alive, and that what was left of my sleep-deprived brain ran interference on my bloodlust.

It was also during this time span that I started exploring the world known as sleep training. We didn't sleep train our first baby mostly because I'm not good with schedules and she slept well enough that we could operate without them. She "cried it out" from time to time, but she typically passed out in less than ten minutes. If it took longer, we picked her back up and tried again later. She wasn't an altogether "easy" baby (are any of them?), but I do remember her infancy fairly clearly, so it must not have been that hard. Our strategy was putting aside twelve hours with the goal of getting eight hours of sleep and it worked okay.

However, what's good for one child is not necessarily good for another. My second would never cry it out. Instead, he would ramp up his cries (like how one dog howls at a fire truck, which leads to more dogs howling) until one of us would break the cries by pulling him out of bed and showing him a succession of *My Little Pony: Friendship Is Magic* clips on YouTube. Even with a twelve-hour window blocked out for sleeping, we'd be lucky to get five, and almost never consecutively.

There were some dark spots even with my first baby, a relatively "good" sleeper. I was still attending baby playgroups and was in close contact with a lot of other mothers with babies the same age as mine. Unsurprisingly, the two most obnoxious mothers I knew were sleep fascists: one who ardently opposed sleep training and one who even more ardently supported it.

The one who opposed sleep training was probably so insufferable because she was losing her damn mind due to lack of sleep, which likely exacerbated her innate lack of tact. When another mother spoke candidly and with painful vulnerability about the toll that co-sleeping was taking on her marriage, Ms. Nighttime Parenting said, "Your relationship will recover, but your baby won't if you don't take care of him at night," which is exactly the kind of fear-based reasoning that quashes the psyches of new mothers. Families require balance and that balance is going to look different for different families at different times. Babies typically aren't well served when the relationship between their caregivers is in shambles.

The mother who advocated sleep training wasn't any more rational. I couldn't so much as yawn without her telling me to buy some sleep manuals. This mother had rigorously sleep trained her baby when she was a few months old and needed other people to follow suit for her to feel better about her decision. Ultimately, that's where Ms. Nighttime Parenting was coming from too: Her relationship with her spouse was falling apart because she was martyring herself all night long, and she wasn't doing it for her baby. She was doing it because she was told that hers was the morally superior way and she had to believe that her suffering had a purpose. The problem with these ladies wasn't entirely the content of their advice, it was also their motives for giving it.

A few years after I navigated those two women, I remembered that at some point I actually had bought a sleep training manual, which had been gathering dust on my shelf ever since. At that point, I was deep into the throes of having a second baby who didn't sleep and a toddler who also wasn't a huge fan of unconsciousness. I grabbed my un-cracked copy of Marc Weissbluth, MD's *Healthy Sleep Habits, Happy Child* and put it in my car to flip through the next time car naps occurred. Eventually, one morning when my kids were passed out cold in their car seats, I sat in a parking lot and read that damn book cover to cover, guffawing and snorting at the more ridiculous assertions (did you know that babies who don't sleep well will never learn to sleep? Like, ever?), and nodding at how my babies have tended to fall into his prescribed schedule without any of us trying.

The problem with writing about sleep training is that I don't have a conclusion. I really puzzled over this sleep training business and decided that we're just not schedule people. But! When I really search myself, I think what I looked for in Weissbluth's book that morning in the car was a justification that it's okay to let babies cry it out. Most of the time during his first six months, my son fell asleep at my breast, but sometimes it just wasn't that easy and I direly needed the freedom to put him down crying because I was losing my goddamned mind during the day trying to meet both kids' needs. I needed that kid to nap!

Everything about baby sleep is confusing and controversial: cry-it-out versus "nighttime parenting," co-sleeping versus a crib. My family has cycled through every iteration of sleeping arrangement possible—oftentimes in the span of a single night—and never found any magic trick (we even had a move we called the Freaky Friday, which entailed putting the kids to sleep in our bed and then my husband and I slept in their bunk bed). Any fix I've ever found has been upended by some development, be it a growth spurt, me reaching a breaking point of sleeplessness, or a shift in what suited the kids. Co-sleeping is a terrible fit for some families and, with the right precautions, a great arrangement for others. Sleeping arrangements are highly individualistic, depending not just on the parents, but also the baby. When parents do what they're "supposed to" instead of what suits their family life, problems tend to arise. Babies need sane caretakers—preferably two of them. It was never enough for a sleep arrangement to work for me. It had to work for the whole family.

Conversations around sleep tend to be especially heated in parenting circles because by the time mommy is Googling "How do I get my baby to sleep?" she's likely already been stretched to her breaking point. I still reflexively want to punch a wall whenever someone utters the words "sleep when the baby sleeps" or "sleep begets sleep." It's a very difficult problem to navigate sanely because it's damn hard to think straight when you haven't slept decently in weeks or even months, but as with all things baby-related, it too will pass. At some point, the kid has got to sleep and that'll happen if you sleep train or don't sleep train, if you co-sleep or don't co-sleep.

BABY PICS FTW!

One of my sisters was a Facebook hold-out, arguing that she was "too busy" leading a "real" life to be online. Eventually she relented, but she still refuses to write status updates and rarely posts pictures. She believes that Facebook is for people who can't make friends in real life. For her, privacy is king and every post is an over-share. Meanwhile, I live on the other side of the country from her and would love some updates. Did my nephew get his front teeth in? Does shoveling snow suck? Does her baby keep his hat on or does he rip it off just like his cousins in California do?

What my sister sees as obnoxious reportage of minutiae, I see as the stuff of life. I want to know if my friend's newborn is sleeping, or that another friend's coworkers are pissing her off, or even that a long ago ex-boyfriend is craving miso soup. These are likely the things I would say to people in passing at the water cooler, when I stopped by their house to drop off a casserole, or when I was doing any of the interactive things that I no longer did when I was a stay-at-home mother. Plus, casserole deliveries went out of vogue long before we all learned the word "gluten." Many of us live apart from our families of origin, childhood friends, college pals, and former colleagues. As our analog lives become more anonymous and disconnected, many of us have compensated by making our digital lives more public.

There are a lot of parents actively using the Internet because looking after little kids can be lonely and isolating. The flood of information that comes from moms and dads on social media is related to the isolation that new parents often feel. It is easy to mock the self-involved new parents who are microblogging their children's infancies, but who cannot sympathize with the urge? It is lonesome to sit at home with a baby all day. It's even more alienating to take your kids out in public and be *that* woman, the one that everyone is staring at and muttering about because her kids are in the big part of the shopping cart having a cage match. It can be terribly difficult to make new parent friends because whoops, it turns out that having a kid the exact same age doesn't necessarily predetermine compatibility in any other department. And yet, relationships with childless friends get strained and people with older kids are often ferrying them around to various activities so they aren't terribly available to hang out at the park for two hours. What's left to do? Facebook. And is that so wrong?

It's quite popular to bemoan the superabundance of baby pics on Facebook, but is it any better or any worse to flood one's page with Friday night drinking pics, or cycling club pics, food pics, craft pics, or any of the other hobbies that people like to document on Facebook, Twitter, and Instagram? Anyone who spends a great deal of time on an activity might have the urge to share that activity on Facebook because that's the entire point of social media. People just share what they're up to. The case can be made that people are crafting phony public personas and bogus personal brands, but the conversation is unduly focused on parents. Of course parents are obsessed with their new babies. Wouldn't it be weird if they weren't?

There are Facebook posts that bug me—boasts about potty trained six-month-olds, an overwrought prayer of thanks to the $150 heritage bird who's about to become Thanksgiving's main course, photos of new sports cars bought in a down economy. Or worse, rants from childless people about parents who "let their kids run wild." In face-to-face life, there are many people who annoy me. On the Internet, there is an equal proportion of people who annoy me. At least on Facebook I can unsubscribe from the nutters.

STFU, Parents is a website that collects obnoxious Facebook statuses and comments by parents, usually mothers, and mocks them. It isn't hateful or mean, but it does strike fear into my little mommy heart that something I've posted on Facebook is buried in the archives. I feel defensive on behalf of all parents, especially the obnoxious ones, because when I'm not laughing at obnoxious parents, I'm being one. Are there approximately one thousand photos of my children on Facebook? Yes. At one point those little suckers lived inside my body, basically as one of my organs, and then they popped out of my body looking not only like humans, but extraordinarily cute ones. So what did I do? I took their picture. And then I took some more. And then I changed their outfits and propped them next to the dog and took some more. Babies don't do much aside from being photogenic. Watching them is boring, but taking their picture is fun and entertaining! I made those little creatures from scratch so STFU, non-parents and *regardez-vous* my adorable child.

While the writing on *STFU, Parents* is generally friendly and forgiving, its commenters are less so. Few comments show any mercy for how consuming parenting is; how hard it is to not be myopically obsessed with babies when they completely take over your world. And maybe being obsessed with your baby isn't such a bad thing since it really is a lot of work to keep them clean, fed, and intact?

An example: I get that most people don't care to think about childbirth in too much detail, but it's a pretty consuming topic to those who have recently done it or are about to, so everyone can chill out about public discussions of birth. Lady bits! Get over it. But I find it much harder to defend the woman who, as revealed in a screenshot on *STFU, Parents*, commented on another woman's birth story, "BEST BIRTH EVER!!!" Sure, she was just excited to have read about a positive birth experience and then relayed her elation with a trio of unselfconscious exclamation points, but then, are we ranking births now?

I am ambivalent about most posts on *STFU, Parents*, but there are few real corkers, like the mom who posted a photo on Facebook of her child's butt *and* poop, a sort of action shot that I can't describe in more detail without dry heaving. I could probably deal with that except that the mom who posted it managed to work in that she feeds her kid an organic and mostly dairy-free diet and thus isn't her child's poop majestic? I feel like I know that mom, and yeah, she drives me crazy. Organic poop. Geez. STFU, indeed.

STFU, Parents isn't making this shit up (pardon the pun). It's a commentary on a real phenomenon. It goes beyond the boredom inherent in taking care of little kids. If I were writing a college term paper on it, I'd say it has to do with the evaporation of support systems for families, which then forces parents—particularly those who stay at home with the kids—to bury their pre-reproductive identity like it was a regrettable Snapchat to deal with the pressure. Because yes, being a parent comes with a lot of pressure. Now that I think about it, my kids drink gobs of non-organic milk. Maybe their craps are inferior?! See! There's one more thing to worry about.

That pressure manifests itself in parents online. As more discourse is immortalized on the walls of Facebook or elsewhere on the Internet, there are growing caches of our silliest, angriest, and weakest moments. It terrifies me that as I mommy-blogged, I left trails of ill-chosen words and sloppy sentiments that could be swept into neat Tumblr piles, allowing strangers to laugh at my expense. It makes me deeply, cripplingly, maddeningly paranoid. If I have faith in anything, it's this one very specific form of karma: Every time I laugh at someone, someone laughs at me.

That said, people can take Facebook *way* too seriously. I knew a lady with fertility troubles who'd get bent out of shape over Facebook. She argued that people should stop posting about pregnancies and babies, like the entire purpose of those posts was to rub it in that she was striking out in the womb department. Hers was a narcissistic impulse, but one that I think most people share to some degree.

My weak spot? Real estate. I try not to begrudge anyone their successes, but hearing about a newly purchased three-bedroom on a cul-de-sac with hardwood floors and a spacious xeriscaped backyard makes me want to jump off a bridge. I'd never argue that people should stop posting about their new homes/craft projects/ finely cooked meals/family outings/cars/diamond earrings, but I might block a new homeowner's feed for a spell so I can cry to myself about living in an eight-hundred-square-foot cottage in a pre-re-gentrified area of crusty old East Hollywood. The things that get under my skin say everything about me, and nothing about the things under my skin.

People whine, "Why would I want to be Facebook friends with someone I went to junior high with?" Well, why not? What's so awful about getting back in touch with old friends? I like knowing who has kids, who went to law school, who has a glamorous single lady career and fascinatingly chaotic love life. It's awesome to me that so many folks I went to high school with have kids the same age as mine, and whether they're Mormon housewives in Utah or working moms in New York City, their experiences echo and illuminate my own.

Sure, I get a little twitchy about the fact that the bitch with the bad Manic Panic dye job who made out with my boyfriend in 1998 can happen upon my Facebook profile and sneer at the baby weight I'm sporting or this extraordinarily awkward hair phase I'm stuck in . . . or—just throwing stuff out there—that I'm raising my family in a rented two-bedroom cottage half a block from a pot dispensary in a neighborhood best known for its transgender sex workers. But at the same time, I have nothing to hide. Here we are, my little family of four living our funny little lives in the badlands of Hollywood, good days and bad. Put that on *STFU, Parents*. I don't care.

MAKING BREAST MILK IS
NOT A SUPERPOWER

I think we all agree that breastfeeding is the best first choice and that it's a pity that it went out of vogue for a spell back there. It's also a pity that every mother doesn't have as much breastfeeding support as she wants and/or needs. However, breast milk has become a bit of a cult. I've heard that "I make milk. What's your superpower?" thing, but I'd like to humbly suggest that anything that a mama sewer rat can do does not constitute a superpower. Yes, we modern, industrialized humans have become so removed from nature that it is kind of mind-blowing that human ladies can grow a person in our tummies, practically from scratch, and then feed them from our tits. But let's get a grip: This marvel is actually pretty ordinary. People do it all the damn time. It is nature's most boring miracle.

There is a trend on Pinterest of mothers turning breast milk into a craft project, like creating necklaces with a drop of breast milk encased in plastic or making cheese and yogurt out of breast milk. Why? If they went to a pioneer woman and were like, "Hey, let's make some breast milk cheese!" that pioneer woman would slap them straight across the face and tell them to do something useful with their time like gather some firewood. Breast milk is good stuff. It has enough merits just being what it is without elevating it to some sort of mystical she-woman power serum.

Sure, breast is the best first choice, but formula is a fine second choice. Whenever a friend of mine gets knocked up for the first time, I have the same offer: "I'm hella here if you want breastfeeding advice. I've done that shit and figured out what to wear so you don't flash more titty than you want. And I've totally dealt with the whole slaughtered, bloody nipples thing. Also, I've done the formula thing and I can tell you right now: Get a dishwasher." This one time, I even properly diagnosed a hind milk/foremilk imbalance for a friend and was actually able to provide meaningful breastfeeding advice that made her life a teeny tiny bit easier. It is the highlight of my advice-giving career. I still bring it up whenever I have drinks with her: "Remember that time I was useful? Let's drink to *that*." It was a special moment for me.

This is what lactivism should be: The free offering of support for women who want to breastfeed and a willingness to allay fears as needed. But breastfeeding is neither heroic nor mandatory. It's an ordinary facet of mammalian life that can be wildly challenging in many circumstances. Likewise, mothers should be supported, not shamed, for feeding their children in public, be it from an exposed tit or a bottle.

But please, can we stop selling breastfeeding as a weight loss method? Please?! All those websites and message boards that breathlessly pitch breastfeeding as nature's way of getting pre-baby bodies back and screeching "BURN AN EXTRA 400 CALORIES A DAY!" must end now.

First off, have any of those people propagating that message ever breastfed? Do they not remember how hungry and thirsty breastfeeding makes a mom? Especially during those first six-ish months when baby is getting all her food from the tap. The thinking is backwards: Moms aren't burning an extra four hundred calories per day, they *require* an extra four hundred calories a day. Also, gallons of water. Saying that breastfeeding burns calories is as inane as saying that pregnancy burns calories. No, to grow a baby—be it on the inside of the body or the outside—mom has got to eat. Personally, I found it difficult to juggle my enormous appetite with taking care of my baby. For months it seemed like all I did was eat and feed. I slowly lost weight, but not because I breastfed. Losing baby weight takes time for most moms. Breastfeeding is not some magical diet plan.

Furthermore, I find it grating that this is the pitch so many breastfeeding activists lean on. It applies not to a mother's desire to care for her child, but her vanity. As if that were the only way to get through to women. Personally, I think the most compelling argument for breastfeeding is that it involves substantially less dishwashing and is highly portable. Don't appeal to my vanity; appeal to my laziness.

Breastfeeding is some legit shit. When it worked for me, it was highly convenient. With my first kid, breastfeeding was a mess, but it worked out pretty well with my second kid. I was able to take my older kid to the park with her little brother tucked into a sling discreetly nursing as I pushed her on the swing. In the early days of his life, we were a fairly mobile little troop. I didn't pump. I didn't wash any extra dishes. I didn't have to pack anything. It was great. If that were the totality of my breastfeeding experience, I might have a different read on lactivism. However, no.

With my first, the only way I could maintain enough supply was by pumping every three hours and then feeding her from a bottle, causing my life to be an endless loop of pump part sterilization, bottle sterilization, and being connected to the pump while feeding her from a bottle. If I had to do it over again, I would have switched to formula. Pumping interfered with my ability to bond with my child and settle into a livable routine. But at the time, I believed that I had to breastfeed or else I would be a failure.

New mothers are getting worked over on the feeding front. There are backlashes against all of the following: public nursing, Hooter Hiders, breast pumping, "baby friendly" hospitals, formula samples, and backlash against all the backlashes. What a mess. What is anyone supposed to do? Get alternately sanctimonious and defensive, of course.

For a while, there was an image circulating around the Internet on breastfeeding forums that showed two pictures: one of a industrialized mother holding her baby away from her in anguish with the caption, "I can't breastfeed, is too much work" [*sic*], and another of an indigenous woman carrying food and water on her head while breastfeeding a baby in a sling with the caption, "Bitch, please!"

Bitch, please, indeed. As noted, my biggest pet peeve with certain fringe contingents of parents is the trotting out of indigenous people to serve as some sort of baseline of what is "natural." While there is much to be learned from non-industrial people, it's ignorant to hold them up as pillars of naturalism. To do so is to treat people like zoo animals for us to observe from the outside and personify with our values, the problem being that to personify people, you must first dehumanize them. A rule of thumb: If you're not prepared to put non-industrial people and their ways of being into the larger context of their cultures, then leave them out of it.

Pretty much everyone agrees that breastfeeding should be a mom's first choice, but I've also known a lot of women who couldn't for a variety of reasons: some required daily medications to manage an illness, others had prior breast surgery, and some just didn't make enough milk. It's likely that the indigenous woman in that tasteless meme breastfed babies other than her own, or had help breastfeeding from other women in her community, but you'll forgive that industrialized mother if she doesn't want to drive her baby around town looking for a nice, full tit for her baby to suckle.

I love that there are so many women making themselves available to coach breastfeeding mothers (because it's hard!), and I cheer the proliferation of breastfeeding resources. I used to think that if the cost of all that would be a small portion of mothers getting lousy with the smuggery, then so be it, but I realize now that some extreme lactivists put something out there that is noxious and worth confronting head on. What exactly is the point of guilt-tripping a mother who can't breastfeed because she has severe postpartum depression and needs to go on medication? Who wins by throwing shade at that mother? Not her, not her baby, and not the larger breastfeeding movement. One of the outcomes of the increasing rabidity of some lactivists is to make women so prickly about needing to use formula that they shut down conversations.

Likewise, the backlash against mothers nursing in public is as destructive. The only way a breastfeeding mother is going to see the light of day during baby's first year is if she finds a way to feed in public that is comfortable for her. Public breastfeeding is necessary, decent, and should not be a big deal to either the women doing it or the people around her. If women can't breastfeed in public, and yet are in possession of a breastfeeding child, then they can't get out of the house much and that is some straight up, old school lady oppression.

Mothers: Feed your baby however you can, however you want, whenever you want, and wherever you want. Any other advice is just noise. Well, wait. Here's one piece of advice: Don't put Mountain Dew in a baby's bottle. Stick to breast milk or formula, but you knew that already.

MY POST-KITTEN BOD

A month after I had my first baby, my hairstylist got fired from her job. No relation, but it was a boon for me as this meant I had the good fortune of her being able to do house calls, and I sorely needed a haircut to cover up the masses of hair I was losing thanks to postpartum hormones. When she showed up at my house, she greeted me, met my baby, and then went to my cat, who was a bit fat, with a tummy that swung from side to side as she walked. "Whoa! Why's her belly so droopy?" the hairstylist asked. "Did she just have kittens?" She hadn't, but in a manner of speaking, I had. My thoughts immediately went to my recently vacated abdomen, which had a sway of its own. Not to mention all the weight still swathing my hips and the sudden emergence of a thick layer of back fat. My face was puffy and my skin sallow and sweaty. And my hair was falling out and creating great tumbleweeds, or dust-mummies, that rolled across the floor and under the couch.

Nothing fully prepared me for the horrors of those early post-partum days. It felt like I was going through puberty again, but at a terrifyingly accelerated rate. I certainly never expected to immediately snap back into shape, but I so badly wanted to feel like myself again that I begrudged my body for not being on board. Though I knew better, I read tabloid news stories online about whichever celebrity had the hottest "post baby bod" at the time and felt like a big ol' lump of mom-shaped goo. I felt grouchiness about my body that I simply couldn't talk myself out of, not with all the feminist rhetoric in the world. I hadn't gained a lot of weight with my pregnancy, but not quite as much of it came out with the baby as I had hoped and it felt unfair somehow.

No matter how many times I read "nine months on and nine months off" and other such assurances about the slow reliability of postpartum weight loss, I felt icky. It was a purely cosmetic concern as I was surprisingly energetic after my baby was born. I went on daily walks with her tucked in a carrier, gardened, ferried laundry to and fro, and generally went about my business with a fully-capable, albeit lumpy, body. I ate healthfully, though dieting seemed impossible because of the desperate depths of my hunger while I was breastfeeding.

I lost the weight after about nine months by being a bit careful about what I ate and exercising. When I was pregnant again, I swore that I would relax about my postpartum fluffiness. And yet, the second time around I was just as anxious and self-doubting until I lost the weight, again at about the same rate. I would very much like to blame the tabloids' obsession with featuring lithe new mothers for my insecurity, but ultimately it was me who sought out those images in order to torture myself. It was *me* scoping out all the other moms at playgroups, begrudging those who were trimmer than me and feeling quietly superior about those who were struggling more than I was. I know this is a gross admission, but I had the kind of anxiety about my body that led to me being the kind of person I always try not to be.

Strangely enough, what freed me from this thinking was the queen of "post baby bods" herself, Heidi Klum. In a 2008 interview with *Marie Claire* she said, "I always think, look at how people were before they were pregnant. If you were a toned, healthy, energetic person, most likely you will be like that again. [. . .] A lot of people come to me, and they're like, 'Will I look like you after I have the baby?' And I say, 'Well, how were you before?' You can't kid yourself." It reminds me of the old joke about the patient who asks his doctor, "Will I be able to play the violin after the bandages come off?" The doctor says, "Well, I don't see why not," and the patient says, "Great! I couldn't before!"

As it turns out, I did not look like Heidi Klum before I got pregnant. I was not toned per se, but I was healthy and energetic and that's exactly what I was after I had my babies. I gained a few stretch marks, my rib cage widened, and my waist grew a little, but I was still me, just momified. I wasn't as thin as some of the moms at the playground, but I wasn't thin going into pregnancy, so I was doing myself a disservice by comparing myself to other mothers instead of being okay with being the somewhat doughy, pear-shaped woman I've always been.

Everyone's experience is different. Some moms escape pregnancy with nary a change, and some women are thoroughly altered. There's no accounting for the variables of genetics, age, and circumstance. Now that I'm on the other side of it, I balk when I hear younger women talk about not wanting to have kids because they're scared of how their body will change. Admittedly, I had the same concern, but now that a few years have passed, I see that worry for what it really is: A desire to never change. But no woman, regardless of if she has kids, gets to never change. The onslaught of aging is as inevitable as death.

Living in Los Angeles gives me a front row seat to the lengths some women will go to avoid looking different at forty-six than they did at twenty-six. There are few things more startling than a face that has been frozen and forbidden to change, or the pinched look of a body locked into thinness by any means necessary. At a certain point, these women look like their faces were drawn onto a mask of skin stretched over their skulls, and it's a little unnerving for a pre-menopausal woman to have the body of a gangly twelve-year-old boy. That's some crazy-ass Katherine Helmond in *Brazil* shit. That look, for all its tidiness, seems less like beauty and more like the physical embodiment of determination. It requires so much effort, more than I have to give, which is something that I have to remind myself of almost daily when I freak out about the crow's feet clawing in around my eyes.

Certainly aging and birthing children aren't synonymous for women: The former will happen without the latter, though the latter may accelerate the former. Hair grows back, milk dries up, and usually the extra weight goes away on its own eventually, but sometimes being a mom comes with physical changes. I will age. I am lucky to age. I look like a mom. I am lucky to be a mom. . . even if it means it looks like I'm four months pregnant every time I eat a cheeseburger.

Besides, as my cat can attest, you can still look like a lumpy middle-aged female even if you don't have any kittens so it's best to not let that fear dominate.

SOME HARD TRUTHS ABOUT
THE VILLAGE THAT IT TAKES

Conversations about parenting have gotten a bad rap, and not for nothing. Because there are so many of us figuring it out as we go along with minimum advice or help from our own parents, shit has gotten extra personal. However, if we all fess up to being insecure and uncertain, then maybe we can back off of one another. This acrimonious parenting culture crosses racial, religious, gender, and socioeconomic lines, but it is mostly occupied by the people who 1) have the time, resources, and energy to research and discuss parenting issues, and 2) don't live in an extremely tight community, be it religious, ethnic, or local because those groups tend to (but don't always) have less variance in their parenting methods and, accordingly, less conflict over parenting methods.

When I chose to offer my baby avocado as her first solid food, I made that decision based on my own research. It was a personal decision. If my mother, my mother's mother, and my mother's mother's mother had all done the same thing, it wouldn't have been as personal, and thus it wouldn't occur to me to be defensive about it. Likewise, if all my friends and neighbors gave avocados as a first food, I might not even think of it as a choice. For most of history, people have lived in relatively homogenous communities, so all this "don't judge/be open-minded/it's okay to be different" stuff is antithetical to human nature. It's a great ideal, but not one that humanity can ever be reasonably held to in practice. Instead, we must keep our judgments to ourselves unless someone's wellbeing is at stake. Go ahead and judge those parents who seem like they're struggling, but express that judgment only by helping.

And then, once we stop being passive-aggressive about things, we don't have to wonder if everyone is judging us. They are and *that's fine*. Imagine if we had casual conversations about our differences instead of silently fuming or complaining behind one another's backs. Say someone comes up to me and is like, "Yo, I don't know if that's the right call about skipping over rice cereal for avocado, man." Then I could be all, "Why's that?" Then they'd be like, "Because I read it somewhere." And I could just be all, "Bro, no prob, but it works for us." See? This hypothetical person and I confabbed about the avocado sitch and agreed to disagree. That's diplomacy in action. However, that's never happened and that's sort of the problem. In general, parents have become fearful of even bringing such things up lest they be given the scarlet letter "J" for judgmental.

The culture surrounding parenting is obsessed with the notion of judging. How many times can people type the sentence, "No one has the right to judge how I raise my kids" before the Internet ups and quits, like, "Sorry, guys. I just can't sit here and use my series of tubes to repeat this shit. I'm out."? Often rants about judgment are followed up with a rant that, irony of ironies, is judging someone else. For example, "I can't believe she had the audacity to criticize me for using formula when she breastfed her four-year-old!" Both using formula and breastfeeding a four-year-old are equally valid choices. Often, what judgment-obsessed parents are getting at is,

"No one has the right to judge me because I'm right and they're wrong." And that just doesn't work, people. *Of course* parents should be judged. Thank goodness children are rescued from unfit homes! All parents have a responsibility to meet their children's needs and not be abusive. Failure to meet those requirements is judged negatively, and rightfully so. Yes, it takes a village, and the thing about villages is that they're full of judgmental/concerned people, conflict, love, cooperation, and generally a lot of prying into one another's business.

Parents can be wrong. One can read every single uplifting article about how parents should be universally supported and we must all believe that every single one of us is doing our best, but there are still bad parents out there. It's nice to have the support of other parents, but it's not something to which parents are entitled *no matter what*. Problematic parenting exists. I'm going to balk when the mom I meet on the playground whines that her elder child only broke her arm to get attention because of the new baby. I mean, holy hell, if that's what her kid has to do to get her attention, something is not going right. Bam! A judgment. Maybe one worthy of committing the greatest parenting sin: meddling. Not by scolding her, but maybe by asking a bit more about how things have been since the baby arrived and seeing where the conversation goes. Yes, we all know our children best, but sometimes parents can fall into a bad headspace and maybe a random open-minded conversation with a parent at the playground can help them realize that they're not quite giving the situation enough thought.

There are a number of "job description for a mom" memes that circulate the Internet with the basic message that moms do everything: moms are nurses, bus drivers, teachers, chefs, seamstresses, cheerleaders, etc. The idea is that being a mom is the hardest job in the world, but to borrow from comedian Bill Burr, tell that to a coal miner. Being a parent surely is hard. And being a stay-at-home parent is hard. And being a working parent is hard. And being a single parent is harder still. But there are always harder things. Let's leave the superlatives out of it.

What's obnoxious about these memes, aside from the endless back-patting and subtle condescension, is the idea that parents *should* be all things to their children, and that is dangerous. I am a teacher by trade, but I teach college, not preschool. Know who's a good teacher to my kids? Well, me, to some extent, but their preschool teachers have far more refined skills for conveying information to young learners *because that's their job* and they have years of experience. I take care of my children when they are sick, but I am no nurse. Nurses have specialized knowledge and can do a lot of stuff that I can't, so if my kid has more than a cold or the flu, I'm going to rely on doctors and nurses to tell me what needs to happen. In other words, gluing my kid's shoe back together doesn't make me a fucking cobbler any more than making mac 'n cheese—even the home-baked kind—makes me a chef. I'm not a chef. Chefs are chefs. I cook what I can . . . usually badly.

There is a growing tide of people who have developed an intense distrust of the establishment ranging from medicine to the government to mainstream food production to schools. While it's true that our world is peppered with flawed institutions and false experts, parents who bow out of society at large are causing irrevocable damage, not just to the social fabric, but to their children. It's an overemphasis on individualism at the expense of community support. Yes, parents must trust their instincts, but they must also trust that they have limitations. There's a surge of parents who are going "off the grid" taking over their kids' schooling, medical care, dentistry, and whatever else they can in order to limit other people's involvement with their lives. The end result is not independence, but isolation. We *should* depend on other people for some things. I'm not weak for taking my kids to the doctor. I'm trusting someone who knows a whole lot more than I do to look out for their health.

My husband and I are self-reliant in that we provide for our family and keep our kids clean, safe, well-fed, and healthy, but we are only able to do so because we rely on a network of other people to help fill in for what we cannot do or are poor at doing, such as teaching phonics and filling cavities. This dependence is a fundamental aspect of participating in a society and having a community. Sometimes that may mean that we're beleaguered by our obligations to other people, but that is the cost of the interdependence upon which the entire notion of society is based. Quick: someone show me a family that just had a new baby so I can bring them some food. Will it be a pain in the ass? Maybe, but it's a freaking amazing thing that we get to live in an interconnected world in which we can give and receive support as needed, and I'll drink to that!

Even as conversations about parenting grow ever more divisive, they are still beneficial if they are indeed conversations. There's a lot to sort out in this parenting business. But if we eschew the idea that what's best for one is best for all, then actual conversations can be had. I was once in a room full of mothers and asked, "Did any of you circumcise your sons?" and I could palpably feel the air drain out of the room. But then one mom said, "Yes, we're Jewish and I wanted the tradition." Another said, "Yes, but I regretted it." Another offered, "No, but I'm not sure if I did the right thing. I guess I'm leaving it up to him?" And yet another said, "No, I didn't feel it was necessary." We all kind of settled into how weirdly personal and complicated the issue was and managed to free ourselves from thinking that there's one way to deal with a foreskin. It's hard because we all come from different backgrounds and carry different emotional, religious, philosophical, and marital baggage, but when we were true with our motivations and our feelings, there was no room to condemn anyone. In that room, we were all mothers dealing with the baby peens we had been dealt.

Most people knew someone growing up (or were that person) who had a cruddy home life, but was bolstered by interactions with people outside of their home, be it other families, extended family members, librarians, teachers, or community volunteers. Even people who grew up with a great family were enriched by their relationships outside the family. Self-reliance walks a fine line with profoundly antisocial behavior.

LET'S END THIS HOMEMADE
BABY FOOD NONSENSE

Of all the parenting trends of the last decade, the one I find the most baffling is homemade baby food. No, I'm not a shill for Gerber, but I think the Beaba Babycook food maker might be the dumbest invention ever marketed to parents.

Please, someone right now hand me a book of "recipes" for baby food so I can throw it across the room. I don't get it! Here's a recipe: peas. Just peas. Just put some goddamn peas on the high chair tray. If baby doesn't have teeth yet, steam 'em or microwave 'em or whatever, and then smoosh them with a damn fork. If they're too thick, maybe mix in some breast milk, water, or formula. Done. Baby doesn't like peas? No problem. Take a banana, smoosh it up with a fork. Maybe some sweet potatoes? Boil 'em till they're soft and smoosh 'em up with a fork. How about some grapes? Whoops! This one is a little tricky—gonna need to cut 'em in half first. Choking is no joke. But that's as complicated as it needs to get. The grocery store also has these jars and pouches of pre-smooshed food that can be pretty handy too.

In the recent history of homemade baby food, has anyone ever made a batch that they didn't take a picture of and post it on the Internet? Probably not, because homemade baby food is all about the spectacle of labor. There's a mistaken idea that affection can be conveyed through work, even if the work is unnecessary. The idea is that parents who really love their children are willing to pay $150 for a contraption that is basically a stove and a fork. Parents who love their children *work* to make their food. They don't just take it out of a package or peel it like lazy people.

Bah! Such silliness. Babies don't feel more loved because mom mixed a dash of cumin in with the sweet potato and carrot mash. They feel loved because mommy loves them. That's the amazing thing about parental love: it's actually that simple. No gadgets required. There are parents who enjoy making baby food from scratch and trying to find the perfect ratio between apricot and mango in their purée, and that's fine. But let's not pretend that this is something one does because baby needs it. Nobody *has to* make basil tomato polenta purée for a baby, so if such optional labor is undertaken, it is its own reward. Baby would have been fine with some steamed carrots.

There is no nobility inherent in labor. Food is not necessarily more delicious when it's hard to make. And while babies can be picky, it's not because they're waiting to be served something with saffron and a hint of orange zest. Try a different piece of produce or type of cereal. I certainly don't decry feeding babies fresh fruits and vegetables, just the phony heroism. It's a cult of effort.

It's not surprising that the current food mania is being passed on to babies. Never before has food been such a preoccupation of the non-starving. I care about food too. *Top Chef* is freaking awesome and I like my kids eating lots of fresh fruits and vegetables. Probably the easiest thing to do would be to feed them nothing but Cheetos, but I'm not going to do that. Food is a worthy preoccupation. In fact, maybe a decade ago I would have argued that one couldn't be too focused on eating well, as it's such a vital part of a healthy life. But alas, the last decade happened, and holy hell, it turns out that people *can* be too preoccupied with food.

I used to live in Berkeley, where I met people who were so into smoking pot that they wore pot leaf T-shirts, had pot leaf posters, celebrated 4:20 twice a day (which is quite a commitment when you think about it), and, when able to form complete sentences, would offer long diatribes about The Man and how he was conspiring to keep pot away from good honest stoners. I was always a little baffled as to how smoking pot could be elevated to an entire lifestyle. It seems like a hobby, at best. Like, go ahead and smoke pot, but maybe draw the line at wearing marijuana-themed clothing exclusively?

I feel the same way about food now. There's nothing wrong with eating and cooking—these are activities I regularly partake in, more the former than the latter—but how can it be the focus of a person's entire identity? I was a vegetarian for many years (see also: Berkeley, I used to live there). During that time, I discussed many non-vegetarian-related topics, including movies, video games, magazine articles, books, social issues, and more. It was not a challenge to think non-vegetarian-related thoughts as I had a lot going on in my turbulent little life. The vegetarian stuff pretty much only came up at meal times or when I had to argue with the counter person at Taco Bell that Mexican pizzas can be made "beans no beef."

But times have changed. While I'm glad that every Taco Bell I've visited in the last several years has been versed in the whole "beans no beef" Mexican pizza thing, I now know that a "beans no beef" Mexican pizza is not a health food, but an occasional late night treat. However, the foodie stuff is getting out of hand.

Go ahead and do Whole30 or Paleo or gluten-free or whatever, but why do I have to hear *so much* about it? Why do I even know what Whole30 is? Oh right, because people are freaking obsessed with food and I can't even open a web browser without being inundated with some food-related information. Even *Omnivore's Dilemma* author Michael Pollan, who is as much responsible for food obsession as any other individual, has grown impatient enough to boil it all down to "Eat food. Not too much. Mostly plants." Maybe I'd add to that, "If you're allergic to something, don't eat it." But it's not that hard, folks. It's just food.

As with nearly everything related to babies, I have to admit that this was not something I understood as a new mom. Actually, I probably wouldn't admit it, except that my old blog is still floating around the Internet and revealing the depths of my new baby mania. I might still be obsessed if my second kid wasn't born twenty months after the first, forcing me to get more efficient at feeding a baby or else the toddler would destroy the house while I was in the kitchen trying to purée a freaking butternut squash. Once that baby got a few chompers in, he pretty much ate whatever "mostly plants" was closest when he started squealing for food. And lo! He was fine. And it turns out a tray full of seedless watermelon can keep a baby preoccupied for a surprisingly long time. If only Kramer's invention of a shower garbage disposal had caught on, I would have fed him in the bathtub and thrown out the high chair.

Most of the cues parents need to see how food is affecting their kid comes from diapers. Too much citrus makes for acidic poop and therefore diaper rash. Too much cereal and the poop gets thick and extra gross. When I spent all that time on the Internet researching food for my first baby, what I was really doing was undermining my own ability to figure shit out—in this case, literal shit, as it often is with parenting babies.

Here's what we know for sure: at some point, babies have to start eating food other than breast milk or formula. Some babies will start ripping the food out of mommy's mouth when they're five months old. That means they're hungry for solids. Other babies won't be interested until they're a little older. Some babies love the act of parents tediously spooning every bite into their itty-bitty maws. Some babies want parents to get the heck out of their face and give them something they can grab themselves. After all, they've been working pretty hard on their pincer grasps. Some babies are so picky that if it were at all polite to tell them to eat the damn banana and stop freaking out about everything, parents would do so. Some babies want all the food in their mouths *now*. Babies are surprisingly assertive little creatures given that a few months ago they lived inside someone's body and ate only whatever came down the umbilical cord without so much as a complaint. Feeding a baby, while often time consuming and nearly always messy, is pretty straightforward (unless, of course the kid has serious allergies and then that is an entirely different book).

PINNED DOWN

I love filling up online shopping carts with stuff I'm not going to buy. This is an activity that makes me almost as happy as if I were actually buying stuff. I realize that avarice is one of the seven deadly sins for a reason, and it is kind of gross to gaze longingly at a $3,000 sofa from Anthropologie for extended periods of time, but it's my harmless vice and I have no plans of quitting. So when Pinterest came along, I was like, *Now I can do this all day and share it with people!* And it was really fun at first. I'd throw a $1,500 armchair up there, add in some dippy dresses from Mod Cloth I was too old to wear, maybe sneak in some precious ornate porcelain dishes that would be absolutely idiotic to use around small children. It was fun.

But man, Pinterest, you have changed! The site has blown up and diversified to an incredible degree. The sheer depth and variety of stuff on there astounds me. Artists use it to fuel their work, food bloggers use it to spread recipes, comedians use it to share jokes, and parents use it to disseminate tips and tricks, many of which are strangely wonderful, like using paint swatches to make garlands or dyeing Easter eggs with Kool-Aid. But holy crap, does some of that stuff get out of hand. Has anyone ever wondered aloud, "Just how many things *can* one do with a mason jar?" If so, the answer is on Pinterest.

I mean, the lunches! Sandwiches created to look like a teddy bear's face with little designs drawn all over it using Nutella; fruit salads arranged to look like blooming flowers with cucumbers artfully shaved to create the texture of leaves; cutting out little mouths from bread and then carefully placing teeny tiny pieces of cheese in to simulate little monster teeth. Ahhhh! Stop it! It's just a damn lunch! Unless these people's kids are a totally different species than mine, they do not have that kind of interest in detail.

Then there are the nursery ideas. Whoa, boy. I'm never going to understand the impulse to hang a sign in a baby's nursery that describes how much the parents love the baby. First off, babies can't read and even if they could, that's not a signal of affection that's meant for them. They pick up that they're loved by being loved. So those signs are, I guess, for visitors to the nursery? I get that people want to wear their affection for their children on their sleeve. It's a big, big love and all the feelings that new little babies bring out are overwhelming, but the signs seem kind of redundant. It's like fancy ketchup. Whenever a packet reads "fancy ketchup" it's never any of that posh sun-dried tomato and basil stuff that they sell at the swanky markets. It's ketchup, which is great, even when not fancy. How does hanging a sign on the wall saying, No one will ever know the strength with which you are loved impact anything? Actually, I have a pretty good guess of the strength with which those parents love their children. I assume it's pretty similar to the strength with which I love my children because parents loving their children is a totally ordinary thing when you get right down to it. Perhaps if there's anyone out there who doesn't love their children, they should post a sign to that effect—a kind of warning for visitors that they might see something unsettling.

Not that I can blame parents for getting carried away. On the other extreme, when I was pregnant with my first, I met a woman at a party who encouraged me to not make a nursery for my baby and instead—*I am not even lying*—empty out a drawer in my dresser and put a blanket in it for her. Which, actually, now that I think about it would be basically like hanging up a sign that says, Sup, baby. I'm not that into you, so visitors know they're not going to see any cooing and cuddling going on round these parts. (I went ahead and got a crib despite her advice.)

On one hand, Pinterest is a fount of creativity and ingenuity. It turns out you can use leggings to make lampshades. Who knew? But on the other hand, it's a lot of work. Pinterest is driven by the desire for the newest, cleverest, and most novel items, be it chocolate-dipped Oreos fashioned to look like a kitty cat, a breast-feeding cover with boobs printed on it, or a *Downton Abbey*–themed birth announcement. While there's a million and one wonderful things about the D.I.Y. movement as a whole, when it comes to parenting, it can start to feel like a lot of pressure. If a jelly sandwich looks mediocre when not cut into the shape of a dolphin and placed in a sea of blueberries, things are getting rough for parents.

The perfectionism, the lust for the chicest interior design scheme, the desire to have the jauntiest dinners replete with conversations spurred by handmade topic cards cut into the shape of unicorns and hung from a giant spray-painted topiary rainbow—it's a bit overwhelming. Like, how about I just hang a fucking picture that I think is cool and call it a day? Here's a D.I.Y. tip for handmade Valentine's Day cards: sit a kid in front of a bunch of index cards and hand him a pink crayon. Want a fun dinner idea? Spaghetti. Kids freaking love spaghetti. As the desire for novelty escalates, it all becomes a little ridiculous. Yes, those paint swatch collages are cool, but I don't really want to get questioned by Home Depot security for nabbing the whole stack of "Open Sea Blue" swatches. Sure, I'd love to have the time to make miniature pop-up books to insert in my kids lunches everyday, but I'd rather go back to the days when drawing a smiley face on a paper bag was enough chirpiness.

I know that many people truly enjoy making special crafty items and that's fine, but it's important that if parents do that stuff, they do it for themselves and not to compete with other parents or to prove anything to anyone. If one finds pleasure in crocheting dragon puppets, they ought to knock themselves out, but let's not mistake that for a sacrifice and a compulsory activity. As with homemade baby food, working harder at something is not necessarily working better. The cult of effort surrounding parenthood—the idea that if we do more to entertain, delight, and cherish our children, the more we'll entertain, delight, and cherish our children—isn't true. One *can* scratch "I love you" into a banana so that by lunchtime the scratched area will be dark brown and delight a child, or one could just *tell* a kid that they're loved. I could hand embroider a curtain for my kids' room, or we could sit on the floor and play with LEGO bricks for a few hours.

Perhaps the most valuable thing I learned in college is that there is such a thing as trying too hard. I screwed up in some of my classes because I was so busy freaking out about trying to be a perfect little overachiever that I couldn't focus enough to sit down and learn. I'd do stuff like type up my handwritten class notes (this was before everyone had a laptop) and memorize them verbatim, and then bomb the test because I wasn't grasping the ideas. When I finally figured out how to back off a little and just *think*, I did a lot better.

I had to learn the same lesson when I became a mom, except instead of learning to think, I figured out how to feel. I used to begrudgingly drag my baby to an indoor playground just to get out of the house. At some point, I realized, *Oh! I hate this!* and I got a membership to the zoo instead. I like the zoo. I like walking around and talking about giraffes, but I hate making small talk next to the ball pit. When I had more fun, my baby had more fun and suddenly going out was less about the very important work of showing my baby the world, and more about us having a groovy time watching the chimpanzees and eating churros.

And I learned the same thing with Pinterest. I can do what makes me happy and throw the rest away. I can use a sewing machine to make a reasonably straight seam and so I make my own curtains. I've been known to spray paint an old chair every now and then. I may or may not have once hand-sewn a piñata costume for my baby. But homemade teething biscuits? That was a mess. How does anyone screw up homemade Play-Doh? I don't know, but I did, so now I buy that stuff at the damn store. I will never make a seven-layer rainbow cake. I will probably never make a cake again after the debacle that left me dumping an entire malformed monstrosity into the trash and running to the store twenty minutes before the party started.

Sometimes I do what's easiest, though the pervading cultural narrative about parenting is that it's never supposed to be easy.

93

It's the hardest job in the world, allegedly. And surely it *is* hard getting up five times at night and having huge chunks of my day eaten up by washing bodily fluids out of sheets, but there is so much pleasure in parenting that gets buried under this cult of effort we're all supposed to subscribe to. I'm not advocating letting babies sit in dirty diapers or feeding them McDonald's for every meal—the work of parenting is real and has to be done (but man, what an excellent "sometimes food," in Cookie Monster parlance, McDonald's can be). Why waste time trying to be perfect when I can be adequate and have enough time left over to fit in a little *Game of Thrones* after the kids go to bed?

Parenting conversations are steeped in sacrifice, as if it's a competition to see which of us can be the most selfless. I don't want to be selfless! I like me. Though, to be fair, parenting does require a lot of sacrifices. For example, I haven't played *Grand Theft Auto* since I was pregnant with my first because I can't have my kids walking in on mommy stabbing a hooker for her cash. But there are so many joys of parenting that get suffocated by ridiculous expectations and "mompetitions." Sacrifices are everywhere in parenting, but they're not everything. Sometimes parenting is as easy as slapping a banana and some Cheerios on the high chair tray. Sometimes parenting is lying on the floor reading the *Hunger Games* trilogy while baby snoozes alongside. Sometimes parenting isn't even hard. The difficulties tend to be belabored because struggles make things seem more worthwhile, but it's worthwhile anyway.

What parents post on social media matters because they contribute to the cultural narratives about parenting. When sacrifice is repeatedly emphasized over pleasure, parenting starts to look and feel more like work, and that's when the sanctimony creeps in.

Parenthood isn't a competition to see who can make the most sacrifices, work the hardest, and make the most adorable deviled eggs. It's hard enough to keep babies and toddlers from constantly killing themselves without worrying if our fruit salad is pretty enough. It's wonderful to find outlets for creativity in everyday chores, but the quest for Internet-sourced and shared novelty is quickly jumping the shark.

SO, HOW DO YOU CONTAIN YOUR INFANT'S FECES?

I don't have much of an opinion about cloth diapers. Well, one opinion: I think it's kind of weird to give a brand of diapers the name "Thirsties," because I picture semi-sentient diaper-shaped life forms that are literally thirsty for baby urine. But that's my issue, I think.

I didn't cloth diaper my kids, but I get that there are a lot of good reasons to do so. I've known people who found that switching to cloth helped with their baby's eczema or otherwise sensitive skin. And I get the environmental thing. Sure, I've read the studies that show that cloth diapers aren't a ton better for the environment than disposables, but less in the landfills is less in the landfills. Cloth diapers certainly aren't worse and they have the benefit of not being made of petrochemicals.

So, it's not the cloth diapering itself that wigs me out. It's the existence of cloth diapering communities. Why do cloth diapering meet-ups exist? What happens at those gatherings? Is one parent all, "So, do you have a sprayer attachment for your toilet?" and then another parent is like, "I do!" And then they're both like, "Yay! Twinsies! Let's be friends!"? Because I'm pretty sure that's not enough to build a friendship on.

At some point, maybe about an hour into the meeting, does the room go silent and one parent just says, "fluffy bottoms" and then everyone else is all, "Yeah, fluffy bottoms." Because seriously, what is there to talk about? A baby craps, then you change the diaper, and then you wash it instead of throwing it out. How complicated can all this cloth diaper stuff be?

In the interest of answering my own question, I went to the mighty arena for competitive homemaking known as Pinterest and did a search. And I saw: Cloth diapers are very complicated. You've got your D.I.Y. hand-sewn wet bags for diapers soiled on the go, your homemade cloth diaper detergent, and lots and lots and lots of Q&As. But seriously, how steep could the learning curve for cloth diapers be?

Steep, I guess, because why else would there be bloggers who use monikers like "The Cloth Diapering Geek," and "The Cloth Diaper Whisperer"? You see, when a parent is wondering how to deal with cloth diapers while on vacation, the answer is not simply, "Use disposables for the trip." There's so much more to it! After all, hotels don't have sprayers for solid waste, you need to investigate laundry facilities before you leave, and . . . oops, I just lost interest.

Back in my baby group days, I heard a lot about cloth diapers, and it usually sounded like infomercials. If I seem to harbor any grudge against cloth diapers, it's because it was so often pitched to me as the morally superior option with careful efforts to hide the costs associated with being a bourgeois urban-dwelling cloth diapering aficionado. There are the sink sprayers, the soak buckets, the wet bags, and, of course, the diapers themselves, which could easily be mistaken for status symbols rather than feces collectors.

To increase the environmental benefits of cloth diapers, one could recycle them, say by selling them secondhand once a child is potty-trained or swapping them at one of the cloth diapering meet-ups I don't understand. But 90 percent of the cloth diapering chatter online is about the many different kind of diapers you can buy, all of the people who make them by hand and sell them on Etsy, and the countless accessories that one needs to cloth diaper like a boss. It's not uncommon for self-described "cloth diaper fanatics" to amass prodigious collections of several different types of diapers. Getting new shipments of cloth diapers is so fetishized that there's even lingo for it: "fluffy mail."

When babies arrive, new mothers are often separated from what defined them before they were parents, which creates an identity void that sometimes gets stuffed with mundane choices taking the place of a personality. There's nothing wrong with cloth diapers, but once they're elevated from something that catches a baby's poo into a lifestyle, something has gone awry. It's another symbol of the cult of effort that dominates parenting culture.

The newest frontier of feces maintenance is "elimination communication," the practice of not diapering infants at all and instead reading their cues to know when they're about to let one rip and then rushing to hold them over the toilet or one of the many bowls that elimination communication parents scatter about their house to serve as infant chamber pots. It's no surprise that the bleeding edge of progressive parenting is another example of "if Africa can do it, so can we." For the parent for whom scrubbing cloth diapers isn't labor-intensive enough, they can opt instead to simply stare at their baby all day searching for cues that they're about to be pissed on, though I don't know how they manage to do that *and* clean up all the accidents that babies are wont to have.

A friend of mine once went to an uber-crunchy mom-friend's house and heard all about how little Joshua had been diaper-free since birth. Right at that moment, as the mother made her pronouncement, little Joshua shat all over his mom and her couch. Because I have the sense of humor of a twelve-year-old, I happen to find that story hilarious. Then again, I'm a grown-ass woman who snickers every time I say "duty" or see the number two bus zipping by.

I've had my own run-ins with elimination communication. I hung with a woman after a Mommy and Me music class who boasted a diaper-free-from-birth one-year-old. As the mother spoke about her methods of identifying her kid's "pee face," the little potty-trained wonder piddled on the sidewalk, getting urine all over her legs, shoes, and even her teeny-weeny Phish t-shirt; apparently a regular occurrence. While few would begrudge the occasional public accidents of a small child, relying on public urination as a stand-in for potty training isn't quite kosher. I'm betting that mom would feel differently about a homeless person peeing on the sidewalk, but piss is piss and if enough parents were running around letting their kids relieve themselves in public spaces all the time, our cities would be even more pee and poop strewn, which is awesome if you're cholera and less so if you're a person trying not to get cholera.

Public health concerns aside, sometimes elimination communication probably works, but it requires a level of devotion that borders on the ridiculous. It's the pinnacle of the cult of effort, with its purveyors claiming that it deepens their connection with their child. And sure, watching your baby constantly to spot when you might be about to get pissed on *might* be a form of bonding, but so is playing peek-a-boo—only the latter can't be phrased as heroic.

Yes, there are plenty of parents who collect second-hand cloth diapers or only cloth diaper to save money. And of course there are parents who live in a rural enough setting to let their babies frolic in the grass *sans* diapers, devoting themselves around the clock to monitoring their babies' facial expressions for a poop grimace. But those scenarios aren't the crux of the trend of eschewing disposable diapers. It's a way for parents to showcase their devotion to their children and the abundance of free time that they have to give to parenting. It's not about the baby. It's about the parents, and that's typically where parenting trends move from being harmless to obnoxious.

THE WARS THAT MUST NOT BE NAMED

Before I was a mom, I taught a gender studies–themed freshman composition class at a university. Inevitably, the "mommy wars" and the question of women "having it all" would come up in discussion and most of my intelligent and excruciatingly confident students (nearly all of whom were young women, because, you know, it was gender studies-themed) would take a side: they were either ambitious or cheerily domestic, as if it all were simply the choice between those two options. I never begrudged them their certainty. I was once sure, too: I was a feminist, so I would never be a stay-at-home mother. I scoffed at women who bailed on the workforce to play patty cake and bake casseroles, which is, embarrassingly, what I thought being a stay-at-home mother was.

I was quite fortunate to teach those classes when I was on the cusp of parenthood. It gave me the opportunity to interview young adults about what they thought of their parents working and clarified something that I had known, but didn't realize I knew. I would ask one kid what she thought of her mom working and she might say, "I remember visiting her office and helping her stuff envelopes at night. I was glad that she wasn't always home and hovering, but she was there when I needed her." But then I'd ask another kid, and she'd say, "I felt like I was less important than her work and I wished she was more available to me."

Likewise, you could ask students what they thought of having a stay-at-home mom and some would say, "It was wonderful. She was always there for me." And others would say, "I wish she had a life outside of me." This was obviously not a scientific survey, but at the risk of being flip, I think most of the science on the damage/benefits of working mothers is junk anyway. It doesn't come down to *if* mom worked, but *how* she conducted herself in a more holistic way. Mothers can be smothering even if they have full-time work outside of the house (see also: Chua, Amy—the self-proclaimed "tiger mom"). Mothers can be distant and uninvolved even if they don't work outside of the home. The work itself is not what matters when it comes to good parenting. It comes down to that ineffable googly-woogly stuff that defines a childhood.

Until I started teaching at twenty-six, I had a series of mostly menial office and customer service jobs. At some of those jobs I worked alongside mothers who were tortured by the demands of balancing their work with the needs of their children. If I worked with any fathers who were similarly tortured, it was not made evident to me. Perhaps I was more tuned into the mothers than the fathers, or the fathers were craftier at hiding their anguish, but the experience did make me wary of what being a working mother would mean.

My entire first year of being a mother was consumed by work dilemmas. I taught for a semester when I was pregnant, and then was laid off shortly before my first was born. I went back for a semester when she was seven months old and then I got laid off again. Tired of the instability, I decided to hunker down and be a stay-at-home mom, which was wonderful, but it meant that my family was painfully cash-strapped. For three years, I worked only intermittently. I published some articles and took a handful of freelance assignments, but I spent my days burping, washing, entertaining, feeding, and buckling and unbuckling car seats seemingly eighty times per day in order to get the household's errands done. Money was tight and our extended family was far away, so there were few breaks. It was alternately strenuous and lovely; moving rapidly from frantically scrubbing smeared poop off of crib rails to lying under our orange tree with the kids babbling about cloud shapes.

I've written repeatedly about the naturalness of judgment and how it may actually be a good thing, but in the case of working versus non-working, there are too many variables for anyone to say for sure what anyone else should do. The so-called mommy wars are some straight-up bullshit and I pause to even mention that such a thing even purportedly exists because of how overwhelmingly stupid the conversation is.

In my case, staying home was not a fiscally responsible choice to sustain. If I hadn't gone back to work when the opportunity presented itself, we would never be able to save for retirement and the kids' college educations, or move out of our damned eight-hundred-square-foot cottage. Now that I'm working a day job in addition to writing, I struggle to, ahem, "have it all," but I'm lucky in that I enjoy my work and I have a flexible schedule so I don't have to miss out on my daughter's preschool's presentation of "The Hot Chocolate Dance." (It was magnificent.) My situation is very different from, say, a lawyer whose choice is to go back to seventy-hour workweeks or not at all. Likewise, I can't put myself in the spot of someone who has to go back to work restocking at Target or someone who is able to leave their kids with family members. The mommy wars are dumb because there are too many considerations that go into making decisions about work and child care. It's a conversation that's the very definition of a "First World Problem," which is what makes discussions simple enough to fit within a three-thousand-word trend piece, but also makes the conversation ultimately irrelevant.

My decision to stay home wasn't actually so much a "decision" as the result of being laid off, but if the situation had been reversed and my husband was the one without a job, he would have stayed home, as many fathers have before and after the financial meltdown in 2008. Further, I was only able to get as much freelance work done while I was a stay-at-home mom because my husband is an able and willing butt wiper, house cleaner, dish washer, laundry do'er, and child minder, for which I am grateful, and I wouldn't have it any other way.

I feel equally fortunate to have been able to stay home for three years (something only made possible by the generosity of my in-laws who bailed us out of some tight financial spots) and to find a job after staying home. So when I note that balancing my work and family is strenuous at times, know that I am glad for this particular strain. There are worse strains.

I know now that my preconceptions about being a stay-at-home mom were wrong, but it took me getting off the Internet and meeting real people to understand that. I have friends who are stay-at-home moms of older children and will probably never return to the workforce. They do it because they can afford to do it, and the arrangement offers many benefits to their kids. That much was clear to me before, but now that I know these moms, I see how multidimensional they are—their whole life isn't their kids. They have hobbies, projects, volunteer work, and social lives. They are not women sitting in spas all day while the nanny does all the work (though those women do exist, albeit rarely, and they're not my friends because I'm still not sure what the correct pronunciation of "Hermes" is).

Stay-at-home moms don't fit tidily into a box and don't deserve the general condescension that they get. While I was still a stay-at-home mom, I was interviewed for a radio show, and though I spoke to the interviewer for a few hours, the quote he pulled from me was my most damning. I spoke about how, though I was currently staying home, I sought to keep my résumé current so as to avoid the "stink" of stay-at-home motherhood. A regrettable word choice to be sure, but there is an unfounded prejudice against stay-at-home mothers. A résumé from a person who hasn't worked in ten years is likely to be lost in the shuffle with people who have worked more recently. I wanted my résumé to always be current, so I never stopped publishing and freelancing. And though I have screwed up a great many things (the radio interview for one), it turned out to be the practice that got me a job when I wanted to go back to work.

The comments on the web-version of that radio interview expressed outrage at my choice of words, but then piled on general condescension about how being a stay-at-home mother is a noble profession. The problem is that if being a stay-at-home mom is a noble profession, people doing the hiring may be implicitly discriminating against former stay-at-home mothers who are looking for work, simply because shouldn't they be home with their kids doing that noble profession? You know, the one that doesn't pay? The one that so many can't afford to be noble enough to do?

Elevating stay-at-home moms over working moms is as problematic as the reverse. In my case, pursuing that noble profession indefinitely would have meant that I'd be working as a Walmart greeter until I dropped dead because I'd have no retirement savings. There's no nobility in that. That's not a condemnation of stay-at-home mothers, but it's a condemnation of my long-term prospects as one.

No one can write prescriptively about working versus staying home. Or rather, no one should. There is no mandate that a parent has to stay home for this long or only go back after this much time. I didn't do it right. I just did it. Every choice I made was accompanied by some degree of agony and was informed less by my personal philosophies or feminism than it was by happenstance. I had to work with what was available to me, which was sometimes nothing and sometimes shockingly good fortune.

The whole mommy wars conversation is misleading because besides for the very wealthy, parental choices about work-life balances are governed by what's available in terms of jobs and child care. If I had family available to watch my kids, I might have gone back sooner. Likewise, if a job opportunity hadn't materialized when it did, I would have gone back later. I can do no soapboxing about parents' choices except for one little thing: all parents should do *something* in addition to parenting and taking care of the house.

Something includes leading a church group, entering your tomatoes into the county fair, volunteering at the children's hospital, or holding down a job. *Something* can be one thing or many things, but there must be *something*. No parent has to do *something* right away—it might take a year or more after a baby is born to get back to or start *something*, but *something* must exist eventually.

For a long time, my *something* was writing. When my first kid was a baby, I blogged too much about the minutiae of my life. When my second kid was born, I started taking writing workshops again, the likes of which I hadn't done since before I had kids. Eventually, I started publishing my work and gaining a readership. From this, I learned one very specific and unexpected lesson. It turns out that a large portion of the people who comment on websites like *Salon* or the *Huffington Post* are stay-at-home moms, the unemployed, and old people. Why? Because they have time.

I often had to wade through comments from grandmothers who were positively furious at the state of motherhood today. Sometimes the comments would include jabs at their adult kids and their kids' spouses, but usually they were just miffed by the whole enterprise of contemporary parenthood. It turns out all of us parents today are doing it wrong. We're not teaching our kids proper manners or we're too selfish. Sometimes we're working too much and sometimes not enough. Sometimes we overly dote on our kids and sometimes we're not spanking them enough. Things: we're doin' 'em wrong.

But to look at this from another angle: What does one want to be doing when their kids are grown? Does one want to be doing *something* or does one want to be on the Internet reading articles about the care and feeding of babies and criticizing the parents of tomorrow? *Something*, right? That's why parents have to do *something* when their kids are young. Most parents only spend a quarter of their life with a kid under the roof. That's a lot of doing *something* before baby arrives and a lot of doing *something* after the kid(s) grows up. Babies turn humans into parents, but parents are still humans. Parents must have some smidgeon of life outside of their children or, as I've learned, they'll spend their retirement raging on parents in comments of the *Huffington Post*, remembering that time they felt useful and relevant and trying to recapture that in any form.

The infrastructure supporting parenthood in the United States is abysmal. Because of the harsh decisions families have to make about working, child care, health insurance, and, eventually, education, all of it can seem so terribly personal and inspire truck loads of angst. It is very difficult to not be defensive or critical of the choices that other families make, mostly because it's all so tenuous and uncertain. It mixes in money worries with anxiety about child development, and adds a sprinkling of all-encompassing fear about the future. Even more maddening, it requires constant adjustment. While a nanny might be the best option for the family with a newborn, it might be less optimum once the kid starts getting a hankering for preschool art projects and circle time. Or for other families, it might make more sense for parents to work full-time while the kids are little and then cut back once they start having to find summer child care and drive the kid to piano lessons. There's no one right way to do the work thing, and it changes all the time so it requires endless cycles of examination and adjustment, which is uncomfortable, highly personal, and deeply individualized. And that makes for mediocre trend pieces, so instead we're left with the imaginary mommy wars where reasonable societal support should be.

IT'S NOT BABYSITTING IF A PARENT DOES IT

Back there when I was listing things that people post on Facebook that irk me, I left out one category: the partner brag. They read something like this, "This weekend, baby and I were both sick and hubby really stepped up to the plate and took care of us and the house," or "Just a shout out to my mister for being the best dad in the world and taking the kids out so I could have a day off." Generally, expressions of love and thankfulness are great to read, but in these cases there's an underlying assumption that the hubby (and nearly always this type of post is created by a woman regarding the man in her life—same sex couples tend not to get bogged down with this particular brand of baggage) is doing everyone a favor by doing what any decent partner would do and then she announces it to her Facebook friends instead of simply saying "thanks." Dads don't deserve to be applauded for *not* going out to play golf all day while their wife and baby are home sick. That's mere decency. In celebrating him for it, the poster is inadvertently normalizing the idea that dads are not obligated to care for their children; that doing so is going above and beyond. No. Just no.

Parents—neither moms nor dads—do not "babysit" their own children. Regardless of whether a mom works outside of the home, dad does not get bonus points for doing his share of child care or housework. I understand that some men are reticent to accept this and that the idea that men are somehow less able to care for children persists, but let's bury it now.

Cultural beliefs about men and children are changing as evidenced by a few of my favorite animated shows. Take *The Simpsons*, which premiered in 1989 and is still—wonderfully—on the air. It portrays Homer Simpson, an incompetent father in nearly every way. He can't cook, he's often drunk, he doesn't always show up, he loses his kids, he acts selfishly, and is generally useless around the house. It's always his wife, Marge, who saves the day. Marge gets shit done and the family functions only because of her efforts. This useless male/dependable female relationship is mirrored in their children, ne'er-do-well son Bart and straight-A Lisa. The show is feminist, in that it acknowledges the strength of women and portrays not just one, but two strong female characters. Lisa is even an overt feminist and through her character, television has gotten some of its finest moments of radical feminism in storytelling. Lisa Lionheart FTW!

However, *The Simpsons'* gender models are problematic, as are those of all the other shows that use the dopey dad trope. By treating men as incompetent and women as competent, it supports the idea that households should be run by women. It's the ultimate backhanded compliment: Women are strong and capable and thus men should rely upon them and, resultantly, drain their energy.

Compare and contrast that with *Bob's Burgers*, which begin airing on the same network in the same time block as *The Simpsons* in 2011. The titular Bob and his family run a burger joint and they live upstairs. Bob's wife, Linda, works in the restaurant too and the couple shares household and childrearing responsibilities. Bob deals, however awkwardly, with his teenage daughter's emotional needs and has a special bond with his youngest daughter, Louise. Bob and Linda work as a team and respect their children for their individual strengths. *Bob's Burgers* reflects many not fully embraced cultural changes since 1989. Gone is the false praising of women for being naturally domestic and dependable. Instead, both men and women operate in overlapping roles and specialize according to their abilities rather than their gender.

My husband is not a Homer. (If anyone is, it's me.) He is a Bob. I suck at cooking. My husband is much better and thus he is the primary cook in our house. I am better at organizing doctor's appointments and play dates. We follow the Marxist credo, "From each according to his ability, to each according to his need." We're a team and gender roles don't have much to do with it.

However, this way of being was difficult when our children were babies. As one might assume, he was unable to breast feed and a disproportionate amount of new baby care revolved around my tits and me. As my employment was less stable and profitable than his, I was the one to stay home with the kids when they were young; the cost of their child care would have nearly exceeded my undependable earnings.

It took a great deal of effort to maintain equality in parenting in the early days. After working all week, he didn't really want to take two kids to the grocery store on a Saturday so I could have some time alone, but he did it. He got used to it. Sometimes he would dress the baby in outfits that I hated and, being the controlling type, I'd badly want to re-dress the baby in something more pleasing to me, but I resisted. On the rare occasions when I went out with friends in the evenings, I didn't leave him detailed instructions. I tried to never tell him how to do his job as a dad. Just as I had to learn to cope with the demands of parenthood, so did he. I'm not saying this was a seamless and beautiful emergence of equality—there were arguments and constant re-evaluations of how things were working—but we mostly figured it out. He's a good dad. I'm a good mom. We usually work well together, except for when we don't and then we fix it . . . eventually.

The same principles can apply to every family, whether they are comprised of a co-parenting mom and grandmother, divorced parents, or same-sex parents. Caregivers must work together and respect the contributions of co-parents as valid even when they differ from their own. There is no nobility in being a martyr like Marge Simpson. It's no good to make up excuses for a partner who doesn't contribute around the house or treats child care like "babysitting." While I'm always down to give out a "yippee" for girl power, no one wins when the contributions of men are denigrated. I no more want my daughter to grow up thinking that household business is the exclusive purview of women than I want my son to grow up thinking that his only contributions to any future family he might have should be reduced to being a "breadwinner." Men are so much more than that.

Treating men as domestic incompetents benefits the man who'd rather skip out on all the butt wiping, but ultimately it harms men and boys by propagating the idea that men can't have syrupy, lovey-dovey feelings for their kids. By far, the worst comment I ever got from a stranger was from a woman who told me not to let my baby son cry or else he'd become a sissy. And though it's not germane to my overall point, I feel obliged to add that this criticism was lobbed at me in a Target bathroom where I was trying to lift my toddler onto the icky toilet while holding my screeching baby son under my arm. And, the kicker, the woman who said it was one stall over currently taking a dump. If someone is going to give me shit, they best not do it while actually shitting. I responded the way any mother would: I finished up the potty business, loaded my kids back in the cart, and then ducked back into the bathroom out of my kids' earshot and told the woman to go fuck herself. It would have been a crime if I didn't.

Aside from that woman, some well-intentioned people have provided their personal feedback on what they think is gender-appropriate behavior for my family members. Most of it is funny and none of it matters. My neighbor scolding my son for choosing a pink lollipop? Silliness. Strangers telling my daughter that she's "lucky to be pretty"? Blech. The great thing about little kids is that parents are much bigger influences on their children than those randoms. The real worry is the messages they get once they start going to school.

Anyone who thinks my husband is less of a man for changing diapers is irrelevant to both him and me. The idea that babies are strictly mommy's domain will persist, but the best way to erode this is to not let it be true. In all my time on Facebook, listservs, message boards, and blogs, I've picked up on an occasional tendency for mothers to belittle their partners' contributions, so it's no wonder that some men back away from child minding. One particular rant about how hubby couldn't master the "four bucket soaking system" for laundering cloth diapers stands out in my mind. For equality to work, mothers must not put up barriers to their partners contributing and must check their controlling tendencies.

Conversely, many families function well with mothers doing most of the household work and fathers stepping in for bonding. In my limited experience, that arrangement works best when there's a lot of money floating around to outsource the more arduous elements of running a household. Some people make this arrangement work well and are able to keep it up without harboring resentments. But if one parent is over-burdened and the other disconnected, then it's not sustainable and that doesn't bode well for any member of the family. Not even the dog.

Exalting the mother as a superior intuitive species does little to support equality, not for mothers who occasionally would like to do something other than exercise their instinctive powers to predict when a kid will poop, and certainly not for men, many of whom feel as gobsmacked by parental love as their female counterparts and deserve the respect of being treated as more than a "babysitter." Many mothers are tempted at some point to refer to their partner as one of the kids, but let's not lose sight that outside of the rare instances when a father really is little more than a brat refusing to share his toys, comparing a grown man to a child is unkind and sends a rotten message to boys. I'll be the last person on earth to snore on about "reverse sexism," because let's face it, the game is still rigged in favor of the fellows, but that doesn't give women a license to dole out the same crap as misogynists or worsen their lot by condoning their partner's unwillingness to kick in.

I have to remind myself of this every time I want to (or do) lose my shit over my husband putting the kids' pants in their shirt drawers, but geez, he did put the laundry away and it doesn't really matter if clothes are in the right drawers. That's not lowering expectations, but giving up a false sense of control over the ordering of my children's drawers. I'm going to have to give that up eventually anyway.

I am no relationship expert, but I have been married for ten years and haven't yet tried to murder my husband. Not even once. Since adding kids to the mix, we've had to wade through a lot of muck to maintain equality and not build resentments (though I still cling to that time in 2005 when he accidentally threw away the pattern and fabric I'd bought to sew a bangin' new pencil skirt—that was just careless). We try, and mostly succeed, at staying warm enough to end a day of bickering about whose fault it was that the toddler drew all over the walls in crayon by snuggling up on the couch and toasting to another day free of attempted strangulations. We're not "winning" at marriage or equality, but I feel pretty good about our prospects for another murder-free ten years, though I realize that doesn't make for a great Facebook status.

I'M THE ONLY ONE WHO GETS TO CALL MY KIDS "CROTCH FRUIT"

The archetype of sanctimonious parents who expect everyone to put up with their screaming toddler in a white tablecloth restaurant at ten at night has been well explored, but there's a new, possibly more obnoxious force afoot, one enabled by certain dark corners of the Internet where one is free to anonymously rant about "crotch fruit" and "spawn" with impunity. While not all childfree-by-choice advocates openly despise children, there is a startling distaste for families amongst many in the movement. Childfree-by-choicers are quickly becoming the new atheists—people oriented around battling the very thing that they're *not*, righteously highlighting their dissidence from supposed norms and incidentally becoming as bad, if not worse, than what they're rallying against. Christopher Hitchens is their spirit animal.

The relationship between those with kids still at home and everyone else (even grandparents) is often acrimonious. I am simultaneously galled by parents who expect strangers to put up with an extraordinary amount of their kids' bullshit and the unwillingness of some people to cut children the slightest bit of slack. I once heard a flight attendant call in to a local radio talk show about kids on airplanes to say that, essentially, adults fussing over fussing babies are more disruptive than the fussing babies.

True, parents can be sometimes be obnoxious and excessively child-centric, so desperate to be liked by their kids that they refuse to dole out discipline. However, as a mom myself, I know a lot of parents, and most of us aren't like that. Likewise, most childfree-by-choice people aren't actively sitting around scheming up ways to make life harder for parents. Where's the middle ground?

Becoming a parent is technically a choice. Though the tim-ing and number of kids is more or less a choice for parents—and having children is not compulsory—*wanting* them isn't a choice. For this reason, I balk whenever people reduce parent-hood to something that is elective or a "lifestyle choice," and resultantly, one that shouldn't engender support or respect from society at large. Yes, technically speaking, I chose to become a mother. Four years into our marriage, my husband and I decided to deliberately try to make a new human being from scratch. And technically speaking, up until that point, we'd chosen *not* to have a baby. However, I'd known for a long time that I wanted to be a mother and when I thought I might not be able to have children, I was catastrophically wounded. Though it defies logic, I was compelled by something rooted deeply within my reptilian brain to grow a tiny person inside my body, then evict her in a bloody spectacle of indescribable pain, and then adore that human who had done nothing for me yet except drain my energy reserves and bank account with her endless need for comfort, milk, and a twenty dollar giraffe-shaped chew toy made of "natural rubber and food paint" designed to "awaken her senses."

And if that wasn't wacky enough, once I finally got a kid, I went ahead and started the whole process over to have a second one. I didn't *have* to, but I had to. And I don't regret it. Not even the teensiest bit. Not even when my kid walks up to me, pokes my beer gut, and demands, "Is there a baby in there or not?" Not even when my toddler pulls my strapless dress down and exposes my tatas to our fellow Target shoppers. However, I do regret wearing a strapless dress while out with my kids. That was just dumb.

Whenever I publish any writing that's even the vaguest bit critical of the venture of parenthood, say by noting the challenges of affording child care or continuing to pursue a career while taking care of two young children, I'm met with comments online like, "You should have thought of that before you bred," or "Since you chose to have kids, you have only yourself to blame." Or, on occasions that make me feel truly grand about my chosen line of work, I'm reminded that the world doesn't revolve around my "sprogs" or that no one owes me and my "semen demons" anything.

Why would anyone hate children so much? Well, a lot of reasons. For one, they can be pretty annoying, especially when they're not yours. But the real problem is that for so long parenthood *has* been sort of compulsory. Some people who didn't want kids managed to escape it, but a lot more men and women were forced to have children they didn't want because they feared the social stigma of remaining childless. Parenthood is not for everyone and saying that it is hurts us all. For every bit that I was driven by my damn lizard brain to have children, the lizard brains of others are driving them *not* to. Being a parent and remaining childfree are equally valid choices, though it seems ridiculous to even have to say that.

A lot of parents proselytize to the disinterested and it's obnoxious and embarrassing to the rest of us. If there's one thing I've learned for sure in my time as a parent, it's that it's too much to ask of an unwilling person. Let's dispense with the idea that parents are more complete human beings. Now that I'm a mom, I'm not suddenly a better person. I'm no more or less selfish than I've ever been. Motherhood didn't magically transform me into a more mature version of myself. I still dip my pretzels straight in the jar of nacho cheese sauce, bite my nails, and act like an overgrown lady frat boy when I go out drinking with my girlfriends. If the childfree-by-choice movement is to be defused, parents (and grandparents) have to drop the idea that parenthood is the climax of adulthood. Likewise, the folks without kids need to accept that they share the world with people of all ages and parenthood is more than a mere lifestyle choice.

I know that my darling "semen demons" can be annoying to some people and I do what I can to curtail that, short of refusing to enter the public sphere with them in tow. I don't expect everyone to enjoy their company—sometimes I don't even enjoy their company and I love the heck out of them—but the tendency of some to suggest that children belong in the baggage compartment or are basically pets created to further their parents' egos must be eradicated. Whether or not any given individual wants children, we were all children once and whether those adults/former children were whipped into submission or coddled beyond recognition, it's not the duty of current parents of young children to be the canvas upon which all that history is thrown.

WORDS WITH FRIENDS IS MY FRIEND

When I take my kids to the playground, we have a deal: I take twenty minutes to drink my coffee, iced tea, or whatever and read stuff on my iPhone. If my kids come up and say, "Pushmeontheswing" ninety times, as they are wont to do, I tell them, "I have another five minutes [or however much] of mommy time and then we'll do the swings and all the other stuff you like to do together." Something for me, something for them. A boundary. I'm no expert, but I'm pretty darn sure that my kids don't benefit from me breathing down their necks at all moments and telling them if I think what they're doing is "cool" or "super awesome." Sometimes they play by themselves, and for those times, I have my iPhone. (Or when we're at home, I have meals to cook or crap to clean up—and a lot of literal crap to clean when in the throes of potty training.)

In days of yore, moms might have been occupied by ironing, weaving, making soap, darning socks, or whatever various tasks were required to keep a pre-industrial household afloat. Churning butter made from breast milk? Oh wait, that's just a fantasy of those afflicted with Noble Savage Fever. Or in the latter half of the twentieth century, moms might have been busy *talking* on a phone (how retro!), socializing with friends, reading the newspaper, or watching TV while their kids played. My mom denies it now, but homegirl used to watch hella soap operas. I was there and I remember because she left the old-timey dial on the TV set to channel four, which was lame because the cartoons were on forty-four and so I had to sit there and keep myself entertained until *Days of Our Lives* was over and then switch the dial.

The point is: At no point in human history has it been the job of parents to sit and stare at their children and provide constant feedback on everything that they do. This is a new invention . . . and not a very good one.

Just because iPhones are also a relatively new invention does not mean that they are "scary addictive" time-wasters. Sure, I play some Words with Friends. Would it read differently to strangers if I were doing a crossword from the newspaper? Like, one of the ones you need a pen for? I also read newspaper and magazine articles on my phone. Would it look better if I were reading something on actual paper?

My little head is going to explode if another viral story circulates about how moms are missing their kids' childhoods because of smart phones. "Dear mom on the iPhone: Let me tell you what you don't see" was one of them. It starts:

Dear mom on the iPhone,

I see you over there on the bench, messing on your iPhone. It feels good to relax a little while your kids have fun in the sunshine, doesn't it? You are doing a great job with your kids: You work hard, you teach them manners, have them do their chores.

But Momma, let me tell you what you don't see right now . . .

Your little girl is spinning round and round, making her dress twirl. She is such a little beauty queen already, the sun shining behind her long hair. She keeps glancing your way to see if you are watching her.

You aren't.

Really?! The writer of this, blogger and mother of four, Tonya Ferguson, actually seems to not realize how many times a day a little girl can twirl. In the case of my daughter, the typical number of twirls per day is about twenty-five. How many of those twirls am I supposed to wistfully observe? I'd say, like, five, max. Like Ferguson, I think my daughter is spectacularly adorable and the kid has got some mad twirling skills, but I don't want to spend the entirety of my day clapping because she can spin around. (Also, what's with comparing a toddler to a beauty queen? Toddlers aren't exactly known for their poise, nor should they be.)

So while I appreciate a good twirl as much as the next mom, I also appreciate a friendly Words with Friends game on my iPhone, or researching some recipes for dinner, or perhaps even my personal hobby of filling up online shopping carts with things that I'm not going to buy. The suggestion that parents should do nothing but stare at their children and preemptively mourn their youth is toxic. With it comes the suggestion that moms—and let's be real here, this is really all about moms—should freeze their personality for eighteen years and dedicate themselves solely to their children because what could be more important?

When the hysteria and sentimentality is stripped away, truly, nothing is more important, but the way to honor that importance isn't by spending one's every waking moment fawning over children, mouth agape with tears welling over the ethereality of childhood. What does that accomplish? Not that it isn't a worthy pastime—there are certainly moments for it. But then there are also moments for *doing something else*. Like Bejeweled Blitz or maybe a little Candy Crush Saga.

No one benefits when mothers are repeatedly guilt tripped for not staring at their children all day. Kids benefit from playing independently sometimes. Often enough, during my iPhone time at the park, one of my kids will sidle up to another kid and do some of that actual socializing whereupon they have to settle their own disputes over who gets to use the shovel and when, or work out a cooperative relationship with an older kid who can open the playground gates to fetch water for the moat. That is the juice of childhood, not mothers staring at their junior beauty queens twirling in the sun and praising children for simply being.

Sure, some parents go to extremes with their phone and social media usage to the point that one has to wonder if they only go near their children with the hopes that they'll do something tweetable, and there is a time to put the phone down and be with kids. They *are* really cute and they *do* grow up fast. But that's not what these articles are addressing. They're attempting to shame mothers for having interests outside of their children.

Here's a quick way to alienate me. Say the following: "I'm so proud of myself! I made some time for me and got my brows and bikini waxed!" Nope. That's not an accomplishment. That's just getting shit done.

This is the kind of bizarre, backwards thinking that has come to permeate conversations about parenting. Step 1: Create a parenting culture that is so consummately about the children that parents aren't allowed to think a non-child-related thought. Step 2: Realize that that's kind of overboard and then get a pat on the back for dialing it back a little bit. But what if we went back to Step 1 and just didn't do it?

What happens to parents who go too long without remembering that they're also humans is they start to get this idea that their only role in life is to be a parent and thus when they stray from that role, say by getting a haircut or going to the gym, they think they've either let their baby down or they deserve praise. Silliness! Taking care of oneself is not a sacrifice. It's an important part of being a balanced human being, even if new parents shouldn't be expected to be human right away. Washing hair is basic stuff and unless parents have preemie triplets, it's really not that hard to fit in a shower if that's a priority.

I know it feels freaky to put a new baby in a bouncy seat next to the shower and rush through a quick hair washing while the baby cries, but it's worth it. Likewise, it's worth it to get out with baby and go for a walk. Fresh air and sunshine is not some luxury that only non-parents can access.

Parenting requires an intense buy-in, but it doesn't come with a lobotomy. In the darkest moments of early parenthood, it can feel like life has been ripped apart and glued back together . . . badly. (Episiotomy joke withheld.) But it hasn't. The sun still shines. The plants still grow. And Words with Friends is still fun, even though everyone cheats (except for me).

MMMM . . . GERMS

Perhaps the greatest perk of having vaccinated children is that I can let them play in mud puddles without fear of polio. Mud puddles are pure, goopy delight. I'd forgotten before I had kids how much joy can be found by stomping in a good puddle and getting soaked with dirty water. The best thing about our yard is the puddle that forms every time it rains a decent amount. It's like a giant, disgusting oasis waiting to be rolled around in. If I'm feeling especially jaunty, we get out all of our toy trucks and get the cranes working on a dam and take all the LEGO minifigures swimming with us. Admittedly, we live in Los Angeles and the mud puddle represents our most extreme weather and it's really a sometimes thing, but man, it feels great to stomp around in the galoshes that we only get to wear a few times per year. I might be a bit more inured to puddles if I lived in, say, Seattle, but in sunny southern California, puddles are a real treat.

Here's my rudimentary understanding of immunology: Expose kids to stuff and they get stronger. Once babies start moving around, those little beasts can find the germiest, most disgusting thing in any given place and then suck on it. Before I had kids, I was horrified at the quantities of snot and drool swishing around my nieces' and nephews' faces and thinking, *yikes, I'm never going to let my kids be that yucky.* But alas, my children are. As all children are. Resistance is futile. And if I thought it was bad when they were babies, whoa toddlerhood! By then, they were big enough to put up a mighty resistance to the dreaded washcloth and face washing became more of a tackling maneuver.

It turns out that my kids have exactly as much snot as my nieces and nephews, and they often walk around in mismatched socks with lollipop drool sopped up in their collars, looking basically like boxcar children. Any part of me that resisted that look as "trashy" or "lesser than" has been eroded by the practicality of letting them get dirty and then hosing them off every night. They are germy, sometimes gross, sticky little messes, as they should be, and I love it. Teenagers getting drunk off of hand sanitizer have probably found its best use.

Little kids get sick all the time with petty colds and then they sneeze all over the other kids and all of them are always sick. Fortunately, we have vaccines to protect children from many of the more virulent diseases that used to be a menace to small children. Colds are super annoying, but are actually good for a baby's immune system. Sure, for newborns it's a different story. Respiratory syncytial virus (RSV), pertussis (whooping cough), and several other diseases that are not so terrible for older babies, kids, and adults, are awful diagnoses for the very young. There are terrifying consequences, including hospital time and, potentially, but rarely, death. But generally, if all else is good, by the time babies can move around and lick gross stuff of their own volition, these illnesses are merely awful obstacles to more moving around and licking gross stuff rather than threats to baby's long-term wellbeing.

Kids will get sick, even vaccinated ones. Vaccines aren't 100 percent effective and so kids can get the illnesses they've been vaccinated against. Plus, there's a few that there aren't vaccines for: hand, foot, and mouth disease and fifth disease come to my mind because my kids have had them. And while those diseases sucked really hard (for the kids and me), they were okay, and once they got them, they never got them again. I could not have prevented those diseases by dousing the children in hand sanitizer. They did not get them from a mud puddle. They got them from playing with other kids, which is not something I'm interested in actively preventing as they seem to like other kids and benefit from their company.

Of course it's a different ballgame if a child is immuno-compromised in any way, but healthy children can withstand colds and other communicable diseases. It was never written anywhere in the human code that one should never have to weather illness. No one should get his or her first cold as a college freshman. People need to develop coping mechanisms for feeling crummy, whether it be lots of parent snuggles, miso soup, or an iPad playing every episode of *Team Umizoomi* on repeat . . . or some combination thereof. It's okay to be sick. I love giving momma snuggles, but I hope my kids don't ask me to pick them up from college so they can get back rubs and liquid ibuprofen whenever they catch a cold. They will have to settle for snuggling on the couch and maybe some *Adventure Time*, which will probably be retro by then. (The entirety of my parenting ambition is that my children will still want to snuggle on the couch with me sometimes when they're eighteen.)

When my first kid was a baby, I subscribed to a local listserv for breastfeeding mothers. Mothers used the listserv to vent about their many anxieties, most of which were born of the psychological shit storm that most new parents go through. There was all the usual stuff: worry about how to deal with nannies taking sick leave, frustration with parents and in-laws, an over zealous attachment parent who was always trying to sell second-hand "breast milk is the best milk" baby T-shirts, and lots and lots of germ talk. I felt pretty neutral about germophobia until one post from a mother about how angry she was that people took their snotty kids out of the house because now her toddler was sick and she was stuck staying home with him. The kicker was she added that she didn't have a TV and thus it was really hard to entertain him. The sanctimony in that post got stuck in my teeth. First of all, anyone who chooses not to have a TV is not allowed to complain about not having a TV. But more importantly, kids get sick. They just do. It cannot always be prevented. They're contagious before they start showing symptoms. It is a fact of life and sitting home resenting other parents doesn't change anything about it. Plus, kids often have a snot surplus for a long time after they get sick, but it's just snot.

My theory about what drives parents to do time-consuming and ultimately unnecessary things like trying to create germ-free environments or make their own baby purées is that it is always about either control or social class, and usually a mixture of the two. Part of what wigs new mothers out about formula is that is seems déclassé. That's why the most fervent lactivists like to compare formula to fast food—fast food is "trashy." Likewise, purées: They show that mom has the time to do stuff like that, and free time is a signifier of social class. Even working moms who don't have the time to do extraneous kitchen activities experiment with adding a hint of cardamom to a banana applesauce purée because it seems like a *nice* thing to do. Plus, it gives the illusion of control. One never knows what yet undiscovered hazards could be in store-bought food, so making it all at home allows a greater sense of power. And likewise germs. Germs seem dirty. Dirty people are poor. *Nice* people are clean. Therefore, parents prefer clean children.

Germophobia walks a close line with fear of neglect. I've certainly encountered a few children in my time whose needs were genuinely not being met. Those wee little nails need to be clipped. Their surprisingly goopy ears need to be swabbed. Their poop diapers need to be changed and quick. These are the basic requirements of taking care of a child, and while vital, are not at odds with letting a kid get dirty or a toddler licking the sole of a shoe before I can get it out of his hand. It's only when the desire for a tidy, hygienic child gets mixed up with fear of having a kid who doesn't reflect well on his parents by always running around with a snot nose that things get iffy. But they all run around with snot noses at some point. I don't understand how it's physically possible for a child to produce so much snot, but they do.

For an older, healthy baby, germs are okay. For working parents, it can be hard to take time off when a kid is sick, but it's also a special treat for both parent and baby. And for stay-at-home parents, it can be frustrating to go days without leaving the house. I know I've resorted to stuffing a heavy two-year-old into a baby carrier so we can get through a quick grocery run without him contaminating the aisles with his sneezes, but we survived. And we're both the stronger for it. Particularly me. In my quads.

There are lots of reasonable precautions to take. Babies should not play in kitty's litter box, tempting as that sand and its "buried treasure" may be. Babies should not play with syringes . . .

even fresh ones. Babies should not lick *anything* in the doctor's office, including and especially the outside of a fish tank. One of the reasons that I'm a fan of this newfangled, anti-industrial-chic trend of baby wearing is that it keeps young babies up and out of germ's way and strangers are a lot less likely to touch a baby's face if they're snuggled against a parent's body. (Except this one time, I was "wearing" my baby while he was breastfeeding and a random woman full-on reached inside my shirt to pat his head and, incidentally, my breast. It was awkward for all involved.)

As with so many things in parenting, the middle ground between neglect and hyper vigilance seems to get obscured. Kids with fevers should not be exposed to other kids. Keep the little suckers home when their snot is green. Parents, wash your hands. A lot. And wash kiddo's hands too. If a teeny baby has a high fever, off to the doctor. If a big baby has a really high fever, off to the doctor. In doubt? Call a doctor. Otherwise, suck it up. Kids get sick.

BALLOONS. BALLOONS! BALLOONS!!
(AND MAYBE ELEPHANT RIDES)

Starting when I was five, my parents made me a deal: fifty dollars in exchange for *not* having a birthday party. I took the bribe until I was eight, then on my ninth birthday, I told my parents, thanks but no thanks on the cash. I wanted a party.

"We'll give you a hundred dollars," they countered. "That buys a lot of LEGO bricks."

I held firm and told them, "No, I really want the party. Jennifer's was so cool. We all got to go to Starskate and went in the middle during the Hokey Pokey. I want that."

My parents responded. "Here's a hundred dollars. It probably won't cover the Starskate thing." It turns out the birthday party deal was more of a mandate with a cash perk. Hi, my name is JJ. I'm thirty-four years old and I have never had a proper birthday party in my entire life. It's possible that thirty-five will be the year I invite all my lady pals out to the roller rink and get to go in the middle during the Hokey Pokey. (Three questions: 1: Are there still roller rinks?, and 2: Do they have bars inside? 3: If not, do they let you carry in "water bottles"?)

I can neither confirm nor deny that my lack of childhood birthday parties has come up in approximately 75 percent of all arguments I've had with my parents in adulthood. However, I can confirm that such accusations will never be thrown around in arguments with my children when they're grown, because those kids are getting parties, damn it.

The only problem with this is that I *hate* throwing parties. I'm just as bad at being a hostess as my own mother was. If you are looking for someone to lead a game of Pin the Tail on the Donkey, don't look at me. I suck. As a result, I've had to get crafty about birthday parties, and no, not crafty in the sense of paper-machéing a piñata in the shape of a giant squid and then filling it with homemade dolphin candy wrapped in custom ocean-themed papers.

Instead, I've gotten crafty in the sense that I only invite very few people, serve simple snacks like chips, always have some beer and wine available for the grownups, and once I even hired a costumed princess to wrangle the kids (a perk of living in Los Angeles is that this place is crawling with unemployed actresses who own their own wigs and are looking to make a quick buck). It's wonderful that there are so many parents who are jazzed about parties and make little marzipan animals and lollipop topiaries. I freaking love going to those shindigs! But I'm not going to do it and my kids don't even seem to mind as long as there's cake, balloons, and a couple of pals.

Other people's birthday parties are awesome. For the low, low cost of a wooden puzzle or two, I get to wear my kids out in a bounce castle, stuff them full of cake, and maybe even get to down a few beers if my husband is driving. The greatest thing about birthday parties for tiny kids is that if I am not all that into the people throwing the party, I just don't go and my kids don't know the difference. Yeah, a day comes when it matters more who *they* like than who I like, but that takes at least three years.

However, it can sometimes seem like my weekends are filled with back-to-back birthday parties and it starts to feel like a chore. For my five-year-old, we have a rule: If she can't tell me what kind of present her friend or classmate would like for his or her birthday party and I don't personally know the parents, we don't go. I've heard parents complain about having to go to too many parties, and I don't understand the issue: go to fewer. I've also heard parents complain about having to throw parties for their kids and again, I don't get it: throw smaller parties. Forego extravagances that are lost on the kids. If making Pinterest-worthy parties isn't a life goal, put out simple snacks that everyone likes such as juice boxes and pizza. Maybe convince grandma to do it. Or better yet, pay someone if the means are there.

Baby's first birthday party is a different breed than all the ones that will come later because it's not really for the baby as much as for the parents. Surviving the first year of parenthood is something to celebrate! It's a huge freaking deal to make it through that first year of crappy sleep, drastic lifestyle changes, and figuring out how to steer a stroller with one hand. It's a massive accomplishment worthy of a parade, replete with a marching band, some of them baton twirlers, and a full-scale replica of the Batmobile. I almost can't begrudge the people I've known who've rented photo booths, hired live bands, brought in caterers, printed custom M&Ms with baby's initials, and organized trivia games that require attendees to guess the baby's favorite food or the number of hours mom was in labor. Almost. I realize I don't get much of a say as just a humble guest at these grand fetes, but I'm pretty much okay with a slice of cake and a beer, and the baby's appreciation probably isn't much more sophisticated than mine.

But gosh, I understand it. After three miscarriages before I finally grew the little nugget who is now my daughter, I was too nervous to have a baby shower. When she was finally born, there were plenty of well-wishes and visits from grandparents, but I felt this weird void left by the lack of ritual acknowledging that the world now had a new person and no matter how much my husband and I were into her, I wanted her to know, somehow *know*, that she was part of this much larger universe of people who wanted her. I wanted her to know that she would have friends, role models, relationships, and an entire messy web of people in her life, but that sometimes felt impossible because my husband and I lived away from the rest of our families and when she was born, we didn't have many other friends who had kids or understood how devastatingly overjoyed we were to finally have a kid after we thought that we may never have one.

And though I'm a writer and supposed to be able to communicate stuff like that, I couldn't at the time. I never told people much about the period of time between my third miscarriage and when I got pregnant with my daughter. I didn't admit that I had decided to give up on the life I'd built in Los Angeles, and just up and move to Tanzania to see if I could find something useful to do. I was fully investigating getting Swahili lessons, and it's not easy to explain why. The closest I can get to transcribing the boggled mindset that I was in is by comparing it to when my dog died after a long battle with doggy cancer. As soon as I walked back in my house after putting him down, I rearranged all my furniture, cleaned his fur out of every crevice of my car, and threw all of his belongings away. I didn't want to erase him—his pictures are still all over the house and the kids and I talk about him every day—but I wanted to make everything new so I could look at my post-dog world and understand what it would look like.

When I thought I couldn't have kids, I wanted to figure out what the rest of my life without kids would look like, but I couldn't because there was nothing to erase. It was such a crushing absence of change, that when the baby finally did come, I couldn't exorcise the ghost of the childless world I thought was going to be mine. I was overjoyed, but it all felt so tenuous that I needed other people to tell me that it was real, that she was going to stay, that I was going to finally get to be a mom. Having a baby is a pretty ordinary thing to do, but of course it never feels that way. Not for parents who get pregnant on the first "try," and not for parents who go through years of adoption paperwork.

I had a mildly ridiculous first party for my daughter: a room filled with balloons, hugs from former students who had been in my class when I was pregnant, a gigantic Costco sheet cake that got mauled before even the first slice was cut, and more people than should be reasonably crammed into an eight-hundred-square-foot cottage.

But that wasn't my ridiculous party. My ridiculous party was when my daughter was five months old and I held a "welcome baby" barbeque at my house with a few invitees. It wasn't ridiculous because of the extravagance—it was just some burgers, beer, and Popsicles—but because of the emotional weight it carried and, consequently, how horrible it made me feel. One then-close friend didn't want to go because she had another thing to go to later that day. Another showed up two hours late. Another had personal stuff going on and had to leave early. It was kind of a dud, if I'm being honest. As noted, I don't take even a crumb of pride in my mediocre capacities as a hostess, but this party felt *terrible*. I worried that I'd never be able to fill my baby's world with the big, stupid village that it's supposed to take to raise a child and I suddenly realized that me loving her might not be enough to populate her world. Sure, it's insane to hire a fleet of clowns, a mariachi band, a videographer, and an expert table dresser, but sometimes parents have their reasons.

A friend told me a story about a bizarrely overblown first birthday party she attended on an actual farm during which all children, even the one-year-old, were given pony rides. Quietly, during the party, the mom confessed to my friend that a family on her block had a party with ponies while she was struggling to get pregnant and she was filled with irrational hate and envy by the exuberance of it all. And so, when her hard-sought baby turned one, she spared no expense. It wasn't about the baby. It wasn't about impressing people. It was quiet, benign revenge for the party she had to witness when she thought she wouldn't have a baby.

A great deal of what makes baby's first year hard is that it causes all the gooey guts of the parents' pre-baby life to drizzle out in the wake of every milestone. Adults who had unpleasant childhoods overcompensate for what they missed and adults who had great childhoods have to compete against their own memories . . . and their own parents. People who became unexpectedly pregnant want to show the baby that he or she is truly wanted. And in my case, I wanted to show my baby how glad I was that I didn't run away to Tanzania and that, as awful as all the fertility tests and blood work that has left me with actual junkie track marks on the insides of my elbows was, it was worth it. It's hard no matter where anyone is coming from and that first birthday can be a minefield of those emotions.

I may still lose my shit every time I see a parent put their baby's name in hashtags, as in "Check out #SkylerRose and her very first tooth!" but I get it. I'd sooner die than hashtag my kids' names, but I get it. All that love can come out looking pretty weird. And that is, I suppose, what drives this insane parenting culture that is currently gooping up parenting, creating meaningless divides, and making parents nuts. We're all just trying to figure it out and not fuck up too much, even as we know that no matter what, we'll fuck up in some way or another.

For once, I made a special dinner, a meal I call "Home Chipotle": a cilantro lime rice bowl with homemade corn salsa (not spicy!) and chicken. Chipotle is one of my family's favorite restaurants, so I came up with a way to make a cheaper, slightly healthier version of their rice bowls at home. It was a dinner tailor-made to suit my kids' tastes and I included all their favorite toppings: avocados, tomatoes, sour cream, and cheese. Naturally, they refused to eat it, deciding instead to eat only spoonfuls of sour cream and avocado.

Afterwards, my frustrated husband and I sat in our yard sipping beers and listening in while our children ripped the house to shreds. My daughter provided periodic updates on the state of the chaos: "You won't believe what's happened to the kitchen now!" My husband and I joked about how she was inadvertently parroting the style of viral website headlines: "What this toddler did with an ordinary bathmat is like nothing you've ever seen before." "It started as a blanket fort. What happened next might shock you." "How this toddler decided to use sour cream is something you never dreamed possible."

The resulting mess was a small price to pay for a little bit of time alone to vent about how maddening it is to care for people who aren't even the teensiest bit grateful for the labor we put into parenting them. In fact, more than not grateful, they actively oppose our efforts to keep them healthy by constantly sussing out new hazards, refusing to eat a balanced diet, and treating sleep as if it were the direst punishment. But as my husband and I anxiously peeled at the labels on our beers and kicked gravel around with our feet, we remembered that we're not entitled to gratitude. Not yet anyway. Feeding them isn't a favor, it's an obligation, and not one that is healthy to resent . . . even if I did lovingly replicate the food from a restaurant they love in a misguided effort to please them. At least they still like my "Home Chick-fil-A"—chicken baked, not fried, and hold the fries. It's actually pretty healthy and easy enough that even I can handle it.

Later that week, my husband and I dipped out for a Valentine's Day lunch when the kids were at school. Both of us were exhausted and grouchy, but glad that we could scrabble together something that looked like a date, even if he did have to be back at his desk in an hour and I needed to fetch the kids right afterward.

We are not a couple who has a "no talking about the kids" rule while on one of our rare outings without the kids because that might be the only chance we get to sort out the loose wires of our life. As we ate our fancy-ass burgers and slurped our iced teas (free refills!), we went over what has come to be known as "the potty training problem," namely that our son seemingly refuses to tame his bodily fluids despite giving every sign that he could if he so desired, by, say, deliberately pissing in my purse because I wouldn't let him watch cartoons.

The waitress, a forty-something woman with a long braid and thick accent, heard us talking about what would happen if we took a black light to our house à la *CSI* (hint: horrors!) and just up and took a seat at our booth, gesturing at me to scoot over and make room. "How old?" she demanded. We told her that we had a five-year-old daughter and a three-year-old son and she sighed heavily. "Oh boy, you gotta handful. And the boy isn't potty trained yet?" We nodded grimly. "They get to that age and it's like real shit you gotta wipe, not like baby poop."

Normally I might object to a waitress intruding on a Valentine's Day date with my husband, but we were pretty desperate for empathy. Potty training is another one of those issues that comes very easily to some children and very hard to others, so it's not easy to talk to other people about. I've gotten a lot of, "Just let him go naked for a weekend and be done" (he's been naked every weekend for the last six months) or "Just throw out all your diapers and he'll pick it up" (the only thing that'll be picked up is a lot of shit . . . by me). Seems like everyone has a quick fix for potty training and we have struck out with all of them during the *year* that we've been attempting it.

The waitress went on. "I bet you tried everything, huh?" Again, we nodded grimly. "Fuck it," she said. "Send him to kindergarten and let him crap his pants and he'll figure it out." She had me at "fuck it," but she went on. "My kids, they are so old now! They're both in college, can you believe it?" I shook my head. "And over the years I have cleaned up so much shit, like up to my elbows in shit. But you know what? The shit is just a little bit of it. There's so much more. There'll be the day they first say, 'I hate you mom; I wish I was never born,' and the day they get a perfect report card and the day they finally say, 'thank you,' and a bunch of stuff in between. At some point you get to tell them that Santa Claus was a big lie and you know what? That lie isn't for them. It's for you.

It's so much fun lying about Santa. That's what you get to do. All that—Santa, the Easter Bunny, the Tooth Fairy—it's fun. It's the only time you get to lie. My kids were so mad when they found out the truth and I just laughed and laughed. I said to them, 'Some day you'll get to lie to your own kids and you'll realize how much fun it is.' It's all fun and then some day they go off on their own and they fall in love and you get to watch, but you don't have to go through any of that stuff again. I just bake cookies and listen. Much easier than actually being a teenager. You need more iced tea."

She stood up, fetched the pitcher, and as she poured she said, "All this stuff, it's about them, but it's also about you and your memories so do whatever you can to enjoy it because you don't get to do it again. Dessert menu?"

After she left, my husband and I were slightly stunned and I said, "I kind of love her" because she just talked to us and told her truth. She wasn't trying to tell us what to do, but giving us a glimpse of how big all of this is—both bigger than us and entirely our responsibility. We've been entrusted with world creation, except that the world we make has to be real enough to bolster our kids as they emerge into the larger world, the one we can't just conjure to suit our whims. Someday everyone has to learn that the Tooth Fairy is a lie.

That waitress was right about everything. It's so easy to forget when you're living in a literal shit storm that this too will pass and there'll be a million more challenges and delights along the way. And it's easy to forget that it isn't just about them in the midst of trying to provide a childhood that won't look too bad in a thera-pist's notebook in a few decades. It's our lives too. I could think I was giving my kids the shiniest childhood in the whole wide world, but if I were skulking in the periphery of their glow, they'd remember that, and I would too. Sure, there's a chance that my children will one day say, "How could you have never made me dinosaur-shaped sandwiches nested in a bed of jungle-like greens?" But I hope not. I hope it's enough that I love them, fill their world out with other people, and really, truly enjoy being their mother even when washing toddler urine off my credit cards.

When my kids were teeny, I went through so many hair-pulling parenting dilemmas, over everything from breastfeeding to cloth diapering to amber teething necklaces: harmless aids or possible strangulation hazards. All I was able to decide for sure in the end was that their memories matter, so that's my parenting philosophy: Find fun and hope the joy usurps the incidents of scrubbing toddler feces from the walls while sobbing silently. This child-rearing thing is so much bigger than the choices we made when our babies were babies.

Yes, they might remember that time I got unreasonably ticked off because they wouldn't eat "Home Chipotle," but I hope they also remember the jack-o'-lantern we made out of LEGO bricks or when we figured out how to rig a Hot Wheels track so it shot cars across the room. I hope they remember my awful Gollum impersonation and the time I jumped out of the shower in a horse mask to scare the hell out of them (actually, that might show up in their therapists' notes). I hope they remember watching *Fraggle Rock* in the middle of the night after one of them suffered a barfing spree and all our bedding had to be washed. I hope they remember not just that they were loved, but that we loved loving them.

ACKNOWLEDGMENTS

This book would not have been possible without two amazing women: Gina B. Nahai and Stefanie Wilder-Taylor. They are writers dedicated to helping other writers, which is not something as common as it should be and I would like to craft them Pinterest-worthy pedestals using nothing but clay, spray-painted macaroni, and salvaged Victorian-era tea cups. Two more boss women who made it possible are Trisha and Gigi, both of whom were kind enough to think I might have some useful advice. For them—and Cadence and Ava—I want to knit little beanies that look like a boxer pup and R2-D2, respectively.

I'd like to hand-embroider ribbons of gratitude to the many, many, many other people who made it possible for me to write this book, including and especially my agent, Jill Marr, who also deserves the finest Bedazzled wreath that I can hot glue together. I owe Drew Smith a platter of marzipan fashioned into his likeness, eyelashes and all, for giving me the idea to pitch this project. I'd like to twist together marvelous pipe-cleaner tiaras for Marianna and all the folks at Skyhorse Publishing.

I want to cook Krista Kulisch the most adorable deviled eggs in the world to thank her for being the first reader of my manuscript and providing feedback that is in and of itself Pinterest-worthy.

I plan to fashion a guitar-shaped piñata for Stacie Burrows and Shannon Noel Webb, collectively known as Mommy Tonk, not only for their support, but their awesome feedback. As for Susanna Morgan, I'd like finger-paint a cast of her bosom for tolerating my incessant text messages and offering advice and input every step of the way. And Danielle Davis deserves nothing less than an actual unicorn galloping in Pantone Coated 7487C-colored grass.

I'd love to throw a mason jar-themed party for all the other wonderful people who supported me: Beth, Susan, Paddy, Mark, Max, Jill, Chrissie, Billy, Brit, Kathryn, Jen, Jacquie, Lindsey, Patricia, Paulli, Benedict Cumberbatch, all the wonderful Child Watch staffers at the Hollywood YMCA who made it possible for me to write when I had no other child care, Dave, Bryn, Timmy (who remains my favorite swole brah despite getting me banned for life from Google AdSense), and all the folks who have provided support and encouragement over the years. And Annie and Joni: I raise a glass in thanks for all that you've taught me.

For B and K, there's not a craft in the world elaborate enough to make a spectacle of my love. For you, my darling blondies, I instead offer my most earnest efforts to reduce the number of baby pictures readily available of you on the Internet by the time you are old enough to realize what I have done.

And, of course, the thankiest thanks to my dear, dear husband who has put up with hella bullshit over the last decade, including the fetching of far too many Mexican pizzas "beans no beef" while I was writing at weird hours of the night. Someday, hon', we are going to play all the *Grand Theft Auto*.

!Kung, 15
#SkylerRose, 144

adorable deviled eggs, 95, 149
Adventure Time, 131
assholes, xiii, 24, 52
attachment parenting, xi, xiii, 13,
    24–7

baby wearing, 26, 134
Baby Wise, xi
Batmobile, 137
"beans no beef," 85, 150
beer, xi, 134, 136–9, 143–4
beer gut, mine, 121
Berkeley, 85
Bialik, Mayim, 17–18, 35
birth, 13–21, 64, 76
Bob's Burgers, 112–113
breastfeeding, 1, 8, 15, 24–6, 45, 51,
    54, 67–73, 78, 131–3, 147
Burr, Bill, 80
Business of Being Born, the, 14

cake, seven–layer rainbow, 93
chickenpox parties, 41
child care, 48, 106–14, 121
childfree by choice, 118–22
Chipotle, 54, 143, 147
Chua, Amy, 104
cloth diapers, 24, 28, 46, 97–101, 115
cottages, 800-square-foot, 56, 66,
    105, 139
cranial-sacral therapy, 2
crap, 65, 98, 116, 123, 137, 145
crocheted dragon puppets, 92

crystal meth, 5
CSI, 144
cult of effort, 84, 92–8

D.I.Y., 91, 98
Disneyland, 3
Downton Abbey, 91
Dr. Google, 35, 43

elimination communication, 99–100

Facebook, 20, 61–6, 111, 115, 117
feminism, 101, 106, 110
Ferguson, Tonya, 125
formula, 1–2, 15, 68–72, 78, 132
Fraggle Rock, 147
Freaky Friday, 59

Game of Thrones, 94
Gerber, Magda, 24–9
germophobia, 132–33
gluten, 61, 68
Gollum, 28, 147
Google, 5
Gordon, Dr. Jay, 35–7
Grand Theft Auto, 94, 150
Griffith Observatory, 3

Hair falling out, 72
homemade dolphin candy, 136
Huffington Post, the, 31, 37, 41, 107–8
human history, all of it, 17

Internet, 1, 3, 35, 39–40, 49–53,
    62–5, 70, 78–9, 83, 86–7, 95,
    104, 107, 117